The Healthy Heart Diet

What is the WI?

If you have enjoyed this book, the chances are that you would enjoy belonging to the largest women's organisation in the country – the Women's Institutes.

We are friendly, go-ahead, like-minded women, who derive enormous satisfaction from all the movement has to offer. This list is long – you can make new friends, have fun and companionship, visit new places, develop new skills, take part in community services, fight local campaigns, become a WI market producer, and play an active role in an organisation which has a national voice.

The WI is the only women's organisation in the country which owns an adult education establishment. At Denman College, you can take a course in anything from car maintenance to paper sculpture, from book-binding to yoga, or word processing to martial arts.

All you need to do to join is write to us here at the **National Federation of Women's Institutes, 39 Eccleston Street, London SW1W 9NT,** or telephone 01–730 7212, and we will put you in touch with WIs in your immediate locality.

A WI HELP YOURSELF GUIDE

The Healthy Heart Diet

Angela Lee

CENTURY

LONDON · SYDNEY · AUCKLAND · JOHANNESBURG

First published in Great Britain in 1988 by
Century Hutchinson Ltd
Brookmount House, 62–65 Chandos Place,
Covent Garden, London WC2N 4NW

Century Hutchinson Australia (Pty) Ltd
89–91 Albion Street, Surry Hills,
New South Wales, 2010, Australia

Century Hutchinson New Zealand Ltd
PO Box 40–086, 32–34 View Road, Glenfield,
Auckland 10, New Zealand

Century Hutchinson South Africa (Pty) Ltd
PO Box 337, Bergvlei 2012, South Africa

Phototypeset in 10pt Linotron Sabon by
Input Typesetting Ltd, London
Printed and bound in Great Britain by
Mackays of Chatham Ltd, Chatham, Kent

British Library Cataloguing in Publication Data

Lee, Angela
    The healthy heart diet.
    1. Man. Heart. Coronary diseases. Effect of
diet
    I. Title   II. Series
    616.1′23071

ISBN 0–7126–2902–5

CONTENTS

IMPORTANT NOTE

CHAPTER ONE

The State of the Heart

Welcome! By picking this book up, you've just joined a rather exclusive club! You've taken the first step towards becoming aware of the importance of *preserving* your own health, and *preventing* the likelihood of suffering from cardiovascular disease.

Let me explain right now that this isn't one of those books that claims it can change your life. Only *you* can do that. What this book *can* do for you – if you're willing to put its ideas into action in your own life – is to help you keep a healthy heart for longer than many of us seem able to. You know, I can't help thinking how different it would all be if the heart was a muscle on the *outside* of the human body. Just think about it – we'd have Healthy Heart Contests (just like Mr. Universe) where contestants would compete with each other to prove that theirs was the fittest ticker in the Western hemisphere. We'd have Healthy Heart Olympic events, Healthy Heart speed trials, Healthy Heart TV shows. . . . But all this is a daydream. The reality, for most of us, is that we take our hearts for granted, all our lives, until one day something happens to make us very much aware of that uncomplaining muscle that faithfully serves us 24 hours a day, 365 days a year.

So now is the time to start changing things. Responsibility for the prevention of coronary heart disease lies first and foremost with *you*, rather than with your doctor, supermarket or government, although all these people and organisations can and should do more too, as you'll see later in this chapter. First of all, I want to tell you something about the size of the problem that we're currently facing, and then I'd like to go on to outline a summary of the solution, as proposed by numerous countries around the world as well as by scientists and medical practitioners. At the end of this chapter you may feel concerned, shocked or even angry – but most importantly, I want you to feel absolutely determined to *take action*. Otherwise you'll not only have wasted your money buying this book, you'll also have wasted a golden opportunity to live more healthily.

Cardiovascular disease is suffered in epidemic proportions in the West, and particularly in the United Kingdom. More and more of us are destined to die from it, indeed, many of our children have already developed the early stages of this disease and they seem certain to become the unfortunate statistics of the future.

Let's not fool ourselves. A great deal is already known about cardiovascular disease: how and why it occurs, why the number of victims has grown steadily over recent decades, and why these victims live, predominantly, in Western countries. Yet our response to this appalling challenge is still mainly inadequate. Of course, there are plenty of worthy campaigns (mostly underfunded) that try to make us aware of the basic facts, but there is no major, unified effort to curtail or prevent the rising incidence of coronary heart disease – even though such an effort would be successful if the media, the government and the food manufacturers together chose to make it so.

THE SIZE OF THE PROBLEM

The United Kingdom has the worst mortality rate from heart and circulatory disease in the world: one person in the United Kingdom dies *every 90 seconds* from diseases in this group. That is nearly one thousand people every day, over three hundred thousand people every year ... each passing minute robbing young men of their future, young families of a parent, middle aged couples of their partner. In fact, half of all deaths in the United Kingdom are caused by diseases in this group.

At any one time, approximately 2 million people in the United Kingdom are *known* to have symptoms of cardiovascular disease[1]. These people are often disabled by the pain of angina, the discomfort of high blood pressure, or by the crippling effects of stroke. Others may develop the disease 'silently' – that is, painlessly and without symptoms. Undoubtedly, cardiovascular disease alters lives, and not just those who are victim to it – the spouses and families of its victims are also afflicted through the worry, grief and financial hardship that it causes.

In the workplace, cardiovascular disease accounts for nearly

[1] Professor John Catford, Ed. 'Coronary Heart Disease Prevention' for the National Forum for Coronary Heart Disease Prevention. *New Scientist*, 26 April 988, p. 28.

25% of all male absenteeism and more than 10% of days off work by both men and women. And a recent report[2] based on government figures available for 1984 shows that in England alone more than £450 million is spent each year on hospitalization, drug treatment and surgery relating to cardiovascular disease.

Cardiovascular disease spreads its net wide and affects us all – personally, socially and economically. And the future looks very bleak: by the ripe old age of ten years, almost 50% of children in the United Kingdom have developed eating habits and lifestyle patterns that are *known* to contribute to the development of cardiovascular disease:

- more than 80% of all school-aged children are classified as very inactive.
- nearly 20% of fifteen year olds are smoking
- four out of five children are eating diets exceptionally high in saturated fat
- these same diets are often grossly deficient in essential vitamins and minerals.

Where once the United Kingdom had an excellent reputation for health, health care and preventative medicine, latterly it has plummeted to a status that used to be reserved for near-third world countries. Yet at least 25% (and many doctors consider 40% more accurate figure) of the suffering and the deaths caused by cardiovascular disease are thought to be preventable.

With this background, why has the United Kingdom an *increased* death rate from cardiovascular disease while other countries are reducing theirs?

THE PROBLEM IN PERSPECTIVE

A 1980 study[3] looked at the trends in mortality from cardiovascular disease in Australia, the United States and England and Wales from as far back as 1950. It found that, in the post-war years, the populations of all three countries indulged themselves in more cigarette smoking and increased consumption of milk,

[2] *Coronary Heart Disease: The need for action*, by the Department of Health and the Health Education Authority, April 1987.

[3] 'A Comparison of Trends of CHD Mortality in Australia, USA and England & Wales with Reference to Three Major Risk Factors: Hyptertension, Cigarette Smoking and Diet', *international Journal of Epidemiology*, Vol. 9, number 1, pgs. 65–71 copyright Oxford Univ. Press 1980, T. Dwyer & B. S. Hetzel).

eggs, meat, cheese and butter. A five-year period followed during which little change was noted in mortality rates from cardio-vascular disease. Then the figures started to rise. Deaths from cardiovascular disease rose and continued to rise steadily and significantly until the late 1960's when dietary habits and levels of cigarette smoking again began to change. Another five-year interim of rising figures followed before the mortality rates from cardiovascular disease began to fall. However, the mortality rates fell only in Australia and the United States – in England and Wales they kept rising.

What was the difference? In Australia and the United States, consumption of meat, milk, eggs, cheese and butter decreased from the mid 1960's – in England and Wales consumption of these foods remained steady and in some areas increased. In Australia and the United States, the consumption of vegetables, vegetables oils and high-fibre foods began, slowly, to increase. In England and Wales, consumption of these foods remained unchanged for a further 7–10 years. In terms of smoking, all three countries noted a steady increase in the number of cigarette smokers after the war period, especially in young people and women. Then, from the early 1970's, the United States and Australia began to note a decrease in the number of smokers. England and Wales noted no such decrease.

Little surprise then that the 1984 COMA Report on Diet and Cardiovascular Disease[4] stated: *The United Kingdom has not yet experienced the dramatic declines in mortality from coronary heart disease enjoyed by a number of other countries (United States, Canada, Australia, New Zealand, Belgium, Finland).* In fact, as mentioned earlier, the United Kingdom tops the list, holding the highest rate of death from cardiovascular disease in the world, with a 3–5% increase in this rate between 1970 and 1984. No record to be proud of.

I had better mention that the United Kingdom wasn't the only country in the world with skyrocketing mortality rates from cardiovascular disease. Israel and Japan, too, began to notice that their people were dying more frequently from diseases in this group. And, just like Australia and the United States, they noticed that increased consumption of meat, milk, cheese, butter and eggs seemed to coincide with the rise in death rates. Neither of these countries had a dietary history which included high-

---

[4] *Committee on Medical Aspects of Food Policy, Report of the Panel on Diet in Relation to Cardiovascular Disease*, Department of Health and Social Security, 1984

levels of meat and dairy consumption so the increase was, they observed, due to a 'Westernization' of their ethnic diet. The governments and medical establishments of both countries were quick to act, recommending that the population avoided diets high in meat and diary products in favour of the more traditional grain, fruit and vegetable based diets. The result was a coincidental decline in mortality from cardiovascular disease.

The United Kingdom made note of these changes but did nothing to bring about similar changes in its own national diet.

THE CURRENT PICTURE

At this very moment, a similar chain of events in occurring in China and amongst the Aboriginals of Australia. Both cultures are falling prey to cardiovascular disease at an ever increasing rate and the reason seems to be an overall increase in their consumption of Western-type food as cultural influences take effect.

In Australia, a number of special studies and bush-land study areas are devoted to analyzing the historical diets of the Aboriginal people. Their intention is to determine the foods and dietary patterns which, until recently, protected these people from the 'diseases of affluence' – of which cardiovascular disease is definitely one. To date, tests conducted on human volunteers[5] indicate that the simple, varied diet of the bush-living Aboriginal of a decade or two ago acts effectively to prevent cardiovascular disease, diabetes and obesity. And, by the way, this diet complies with dietary recommendations, made in many · countries, designed to reduce mortality from cardiovascular disease.

And in China, the party leader Mr. Zhao Ziyang addressing delegates at the National People's Congress (April 1988) warned that China must learn a lesson from the errors of developed countries and prevent over-consumption of meat, fish and eggs. Furthermore, Mr. Zhao warned, action must be taken urgently to create a new food pattern with Chinese characteristics' in order to prevent widespread obesity, diabetes and cardiovascular disease among China's 1.8 billion people.

Mr. Zhao is not alone in his support of the more traditional diet. Researchers from the United States, China and England

[5] 'The Healthiest Restaurant in Australia' Stephanie Pain, *New Scientist*, 18 August 1988, pg 42.

are presently completing a six-year study[6] of Chinese dietary patterns which gives strong indications that the 'diseases of affluence' may be easily avoided by following a traditional Chinese diet. Although this diet is high in calories from complex carbohydrates, it is significantly low in fat and cholesterol, and very high in fibre – just what Western medicine currently recommends as a diet to prevent cardiovascular disease.

In Western terms, Mr. Zhao's recommendations are the epitome of preventative action for he is considering solutions to problems that could evolve, on a massive scale, over the next ten to thirty years unless corrective measures are taken immediately.

Here in the United Kingdom, however, death from cardiovascular disease is stll on the increase.

THE MEASURE OF PREVENTION

Why have death rates from coronary heart disease fallen, since 1970, in many countries in the Western world? The United States and many European countries have reduced their mortality rates by 30% *or more* since this time. Their strategy, almost without exception, has been to take swift preventative action on a national scale.

The prevention, reduction and sometimes reversal of cardiovascular disease is achieved by addressing three main areas of lifestyle:

- Diet: a reduction of saturated fats, salt and low-fibre foods
- Exercise: an increase in exercise for all ages
- Smoking: a reduction in smoking, especially of cigarettes

In countries where large-scale prevention is successful, these actions are supported at several levels in the social, governmental and economic intra-structures. This is a summary of how and where such support is achieved:

- Health education for all age groups, from young school children to old age pensioners, on the detrimental effects of smoking, lack of exercise and poor diet, with emphasis on how to achieve a healthy diet.
- Additional education in these areas for doctors, teachers and other professionals whose opinions affect the lifestyles of large numbers of people.

[6] T. Colin Campbell, Cornell University; Chen Junshi, Chinese Academy of Preventive Medicine; Li Jungao, Chinese Academy of Medical Sciences; Richard Peto, Oxford University (full report to be published in 1989).

- Significant funding for continued research into and monitoring of the prevention, reduction and treatment of cardiovascular disease.
- Use of mass media to reinforce these positive health messages.
- Government legislation to exert pressure on cigarette and food manufacturers so that they comply with labelling and manufacturing regulations.
- Social, governmental and media pressure on food manufacturers to meet public demand for healthy, nutritionally adequate food products.
- Social and governmental pressure on schools, places of work and other public organisations to supply facilities for exercise and adequate health monitoring programmes.
- Economic incentive – through insurance and pension schemes, for instance – to achieve healthy standards of lifestyle.

Countries which have met all or several of these standards have enjoyed significant reduction in their mortality rates from coronary heart disease and an overall improvement in the health of their population. In short, *preventative action works* and, as these countries have proved, it works on a national scale over a long period of time. Though proof of this nature is now abundant (twelve of the fifteen countries previously at the top of the cardiovascular disease list have reduced their mortality rates), the United Kingdom continues to drag its medical, economic and political heels. Where other countries are saving lives, too many people who should know better in the United Kingdom are *still* discussing whether or not diet, smoking and exercise can make a difference!

Why is the United Kingdom lagging so dreadfully far behind? A large measure of responsibility must rest on the shoulders of those scientists, governmental advisors, and representatives of certain food manufacturers who seem to have conspired to bring about a state of no-change. In 1974 the Department of Health and Social Security published the report *Diet and Coronary Heart Disease*, assembled by an advisory panel to the Committee on Medical Aspects of Food Policy (COMA). Although medical reports from other countries, as well as the World Health Organisation, made virtually unanimous recommendations that certain dietary patterns, particularly high levels of saturated fats in the diet, were to blame for high mortality rates from cardiovascular disease, the 1974 COMA report stated that its panel was:

'. . . unconvinced by the available evidence that the incidence of coronary heart disease in the United Kingdom, or the death rate from it, would be reduced in consequence of a rise in the ratio of polyunsaturated to saturated fatty acids in the national diet.'

The report concluded that:

'in the context of the United Kingdom diet, claims that eating or not eating a particular type of food could reduce the risk of coronary heart disease were completely unjustified.'

Then in 1976, a group of doctors from the Royal College of Physicians got together with a panel from the British Cardiac Society and published a report entitled *The Prevention of Coronary Heart Disease*, which recommended a reduction in the dietary intake of saturated fats. In 1977 the Committee on Medical Aspects of Food Policy (COMA) reconsidered their 1974 report and again endorsed its recommendations, thus establishing a clear difference between medical and government motives, one that has not yet been reconciled.

Nine years after the first COMA report, the National Advisory Committee on Nutrition Education (NACNE) published its own report. The committee was comprised of working parties from government, medical and food organisations; the report was commissioned by the Department of Health and Social Security in order to develop national dietary goals and guidelines. It recommended:

- a 25% reduction in total fat consumption
- a 40% reduction in saturated fat consumption
- a 50% reduction in sugar consumption
- a 50% increase in dietary fibre
- a general reduction in alcohol consumption

This, at least, was a step in the right direction, albeit a painfully slow one. Nevertheless, government officials (particularly those with close links to certain food industries), as well as those food industries most likely to be affected by the implications of the report immediately condemned it. Some of these threatened industries even started to put out their own counter-propaganda – the meat industry, for example, hired its own expert nutritionist, as the headline in the Meat Trades Journal made clear: 'Top nutritionist joins forces with the Meat Promotion Executive to *quash the health lobby*'![7] It is rare, I think, for any

[7] *Meat Trades Journal*, June 28th 1984.

industry to so openly acknowledge its outright opposition to the spread of healthy eating habits.

The rationale of opposition to these changes towards a more healthy diet is built around the words 'conclusive proof'. Just what *is* 'conclusive proof'? As long as *one* person somewhere is able to eat an unhealthy diet and get away with it, then the proof that an unhealthy diet leads to coronary heart disease cannot be called 'conclusive'. And as long as there is *one* scientist or nutritionist (frequently no more than a paid industry spokesman) who is prepared to voice his dissent in public, then the proof cannot be called 'conclusive'. Although you and I may consider this to be no more than playing with words, this line of reasoning was central to the next COMA report, issued ten years after the first one. In it, the recommendations of the NACNE report were significantly reduced, on the basis that *'we doubt whether the stringent dietary changes ... would be implemented by the general population at the present time.'* The panel further stated that, although it had considered *'the complex relationship between diet and cardiovascular disease'*, it found that *'the evidence falls short of proof.'* The COMA Panel finally *declined to prescribe a national diet.* Another wasted opportunity.

Amongst developed countries, Britain now had one of the lowest expectations of longevity past the age of forty-five. Meanwhile, in America, the National Institutes of Health launched a campaign to reform the American diet in order to reduce cholesterol levels in the blood, and thereby reduce the incidence of cardiovascular disease. Simultaneously, the European Atherosclerosis Society announced recommendations regarding acceptable and excessive levels of cholesterol in the blood. Its recommendations were studied by Barry Lewis of St. Thomas's Hospital in London who concluded that '50% of us [in Britain] have levels [of cholesterol] above those recommended.'

Yet, when the Nutrition Society met in London in mid-July (1986) a number of its members still proposed the point of view that there was not yet a *proven* link between diet and heart disease. But, as Basil Rifkind of the American National Institutes of Health pointed out: 'We will never have the luxury of a completely satisfactory study that diet is linked to coronary heart disease. . . .' He was supported by Geoffrey Rose, an epidemiologist from the London School of Hygiene and Tropical Medicine, who said ' ... there can be no proof, except by hindsight.' Both Rose and Rifkind expressed the need to act upon the knowledge available to save lives rather than wait years, possibly decades, for the conclusive proof that so many people seemed to be waiting for.

As one remarkably sensible expert, Dr. Jim Mann of the Department of Community Medicine and General Practice, Radcliffe Infirmary, Oxford put it: 'There are lots of reasons for saying that a low fat, high fibre diet is healthier, but the arguments for the prevention of heart disease are the strongest. I think some commentators have done the country a great disservice by saying that fat intake levels is an area of controversy, in fact there is no controversy and if we followed the example of the united States, Finland and Australia we would get the same benefit.' In April 1988 the National Forum for Coronary Heart Disease Prevention published a report entitled simply *Coronary Heart Disease Prevention*. The report highlights several shortcomings of our official atttude towards coronary heart disease prevention, not least the *Look After Your Heart Campaign* which the Health Education Authority launched in 1987. This campaign is described as 'woefully inadequate'. Other criticisms and recomendations include:

- A DHSS system to monitor, on a national scale, the prevalence of major risk factors for coronary heart disease.
- A Government ban on tobacco advertising and sports sponsorship, as well as increased taxes on tobacco.
- More government funds into research for treatment and prevention of coronary heart disease.
- Statutory labelling regulations for the nutritional aspects of all food products.
- Non-commercial health education for school children.
- Government funding for national promotion of sports and exercise (note: the government *cut* funding to the Sports Council by £3 million in 1987).
- More resources for health practitioners to test and monitor individuals and communities, including equipment to measure levels of cholesterol in the blood.

Clearly the Forum is less than impressed with government action. Anne Dillon, Director of the Coronary Prevention Group – just one of the thirty organisations in the Forum – summarised the Forum's wishes when she said '*We seek a national policy that underpins rather than undermines health messages.*'

LEFT TO OUR OWN FATE

In the 1980's over two and a half million people have died from cardiovascular disease in Great Britain. If, as was suggested earlier, just one quarter of these deaths could have been avoided by application of current preventative measures, then 600,000 cardiovascular disease victims might still be with us. And remember, some scientists think the figure of preventable deaths could be closer to 40% – that means that a shocking 120,000 deaths *each year* could have been avoided.

The probability is high that one of those victims of coronary heart disease was a friend of yours – maybe an acquaintance, maybe someone you worked with. One of those victims might have been someone you knew and loved. One more person who just might – if he or she had been given the chance – still be with us.

I suggest that it is up to each one of us to address the whole question of cardiovascular disease, as it affects our own lives. Heart disease is everyone's problem but, more particularly, it is *your* problem – until, that is, you've taken steps to gather the available facts and recommendations, and then learnt how to apply them to your own lifestyle and diet. This is the only way – *the only way* – that we can begin to protect ourselves, our families and our children from the epidemic of cardiovascular disease that is currently raging – all too unchallenged – in the United Kingdom.

CHAPTER TWO

What Makes You Tick?

Wherever you are and whatever you happen to be doing at any time of the day or night, your body is silently busy performing all of the tasks necessary to keep you alive. Of course, you are familiar with the outward processes such as eating, breathing, excreting and sleeping which are essential life-sustaining functions, but even more basic than these are the processes of life that occur at a cellular level. That is, each and every cell in your body is subject to needs and events that remain hidden from view but which, nonetheless, lay the foundations for your health.

THE CARDIOVASCULAR SYSTEM

Every living cell in your body has a specific job to do and in order that each cell may do its job well, it must somehow take essential products in and put waste material out. In addition, it is very important that there is neither a surplus of essential products, nor a build-up of waste materials to interfere with the efficient working of individual cells. To meet this requirement, the cells of your body need a reliable transport system that will perform both deliveries and removals. The circulation of blood is such a system. It is called the cardiovascular system because it is structured around the heart (cardio) and the blood vessels (vascular) and all the functions included in the relationship between them.

BLOOD

Let's start with the blood and look at how it is made up so that we can understand its value and importance.

Blood is composed of red cells, white cells and platelets suspended in plasma – if you've ever made a salad dressing from vinegar, oil and a few herbs you'll understand the idea of suspension. When you stir the mixture, it changes in consistency and, temporarily at least, the oil, vinegar and herbs are evenly .

distributed, making a smooth emulsion. Blood is, in analogy only, a similar mixture. All four components – plasma, platelets, red and white cells – are present in measured and changing proportions to make healthy blood. Let's look, briefly, at each of its components.

PLASMA

If any substance on earth could be called primordial soup, it would have to be plasma. To make it, take several litres of water and add microscopic portions of several dozen compounds such as amino acids, hormones, antibodies, 'tissue salts' such as sodium, potassium, calcium and chloride, and proteins such as albumin, globulin and fibrinogen.

These nutrients are transferred to your needy cells in exchange for waste materials for eventual excretion. Here's how: every cell in your body is surrounded by a plasma-like liquid called tissue fluid. This fluid gets right up next to the cell, every cell, and removes any waste material that the cell generates as it functions. This waste is transferred through the tissue fluid to the plasma and, at this point, is exchanged for whichever of the compounds in the plasma the needy cell requires. These compounds are transferred from the plasma, through the tissue fluid to the waiting body cell. The only difference is that this whole cycle happens about one-hundred times faster than it took you to read about it!

RED BLOOD CELLS

These cells (also called erythrocytes) are suspended in your plasma. They are red because they contain a red pigment, called haemoglobin, which has a little bit of iron in its centre. However, haemoglobin doesn't only colour your blood red, it is the aspect of each red blood cell that enables that cell to carry oxygen and transfer it, eventually, to your body tissues.

In conditions where there is a high concentration of oxygen, such as in your lungs, haemoglobin actually combines with oxygen. Then, when that red blood cell moves into the reverse conditions of low concentration of oxygen, such as tissue in your limbs, it releases its oxygen. In other words, the oxygen is transferred from the red blood cell to the needy tissues.

WHITE BLOOD CELLS

Also called leucocytes, these cells are much larger in size than the red blood cells, but there is only one white cell to every five or six hundred red, depending on where they are measured in your body. The white blood cells come in three forms, each with its distinct function, but their collective purpose is to destroy or protect you from foreign organisms such as 'germs', viruses and bacteria. So next time you cut your finger, give a special thought to those white blood cells which are rapidly gathering at the site to carry off dead tissue and destroy invading bactria.

PLATELETS

These are tiny cells that are present to help in the process of clotting. They are necessary in order for fibrinogen (a protein in your plasma) to convert to fibrin. Fibrin forms into fine threads which surround the blood cells and then contract to form them into an ever more solid mass – a blood clot.

In summary, the function of your blood is to use its component parts to protect your body tissues and to transport substances to and from the tissue cells.

Protection is gained from:

- the salts, contained in your plasma, which provide a safe, appropriate environment for living cells
- the white blood cells which fight off bacteria and invading organisms and converge at the site of wounds
- the fibrinogen in your plasma which converts to fibrin and causes blood to clot at the side of wounds.

The *transport* function of the blood is to:

- carry food nutrients to the tissues from the digestive system
- carry oxygen from the lungs to the tissues
- carry hormones from the glands that supply them to the tissues that need them
- carry white blood cells to points in the body that require their protective action
- carry waste materials from the tissues to their point of excretion
- regulate body temperature by transferring heat from active to less active tissues, or to the skin surface for removal.

The average man has five to six litres of blood in his body at any one time, the average woman has four to five litres. In order for this wonderful liquid to do its work, however, it needs to move around the body, to circulate.

Your body achieves circulation of the blood in a fairly mechanical way using a pump, a network of channels and a variety of valves. Let's look at each aspect of this circulation.

HEART

Your heart is a small, msucular sac about the size of your clenched fist. It is located in a fairly central position in your body – just behind and slightly to the left of your breastbone so that its pumping action is performed efficiently. Your heart pumps blood to every part of your body between sixty and ninety times each minute, every day of your life, just by contracting its muscles. Let's look inside the heart to see how it is made and precisely what is happening as it pumps.

A thick wall divides the inside of your heart into two completely separate halves, left and right. Within each of these halves are two further divisions – the top chambers, called atria, and the bottom chambers, called ventricles.

The top chambers, atria, have thin walls of muscle and these

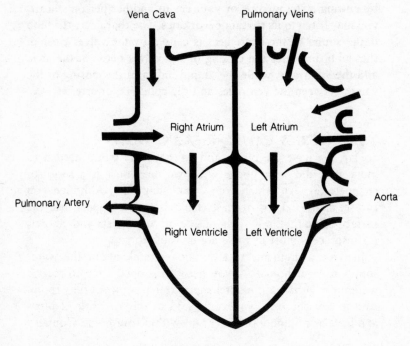

chambers act as 'waiting rooms' for the blood that enters them. Once the blood enters the atrium it cannot leave except by passing through a valve, a sort of one-way door, into the lower chamber. This door only opens when it is forced: the muscular walls of the atrium contract and push the blood against the valve causing it to open and allowing the blood to flow through into the lower chamber.

The lower chamber in each half of your heart is called a ventricle. The ventricles have thick walls of muscle because these chambers have to work harder than the atria. Once blood is pushed out of the atria and into the ventricles it cannot return to the upper chamber (remember, that valve was one-way). Instead, it will be pushed out of the ventricle, through another one-way valve, into a narrow conduit. This conduit will channel the blood to a number of destinations in your body – your toes, your fingertips, your lungs, your brain. Wherever it is going, it will need a very strong push to *keep* it going. The initial push given to that blood occurs when the muscles of each ventricle contract. Now you can see why the muscle walls of these chambers are thicker than those of the atria.

This transfer of blood from the atria to the ventricles takes place in a rhythmic cycle every moment of your life. By and large, one remains unaware of this cycle but, after exertion or by putting a stethoscope or your ear to another person's heart, you may listen to its rhythmic workings. The characteristic 'lubb dupp' sound of the heart beat is caused by the valves closing: the 'lubb' indicates the closing of the valves between the atria and the ventricles, while the 'dupp' indicates the closing of the valves between the ventricles and the conduits, or arteries.

THE ARTERIES, CAPILLARIES AND VEINS

So far, we have the blood and we have the pump needed to move it round your body. What we need now is a series of channels through which your blood may flow. Although you can see signs of a few of these channels as they appear near the surface of your skin – at the inside of your wrists and elbows, for instance – most of these are invisible to you.

Just for a moment, as an analogy, think about the water supply to your home. All you need do is open a tap to receive water in your bathroom, kitchen, central heating or utility room. And if you chose to, you could add to this network of pipes and have any number of water taps within your home. You also have another network of pipes in your home that takes used water away – drains. This combination of water pipes and drains means that you have continuous access to water and an efficient means of putting surplus or used water back into the circulating water system.

In a network similar to the water system in your home, the heart and blood rely on narrow conduits in your body which contain your blood and channel it towards a specific location in your body with speed and precision. There are three basic types of channels or conduits for your blood: the arteries, the capillaries and the veins. This is how they work.

THE ARTERIES

Arteries are the conduits that channel blood away from your heart to the limbs and organs. Arteries are round tubes constructed in three layers. The outer layer is tough and fibrous to protect the artery and give it strength. The middle layer is predominantly muscle tissue, with a small number of elastic fibres. This combination gives the artery flexibility as well as the ability to adjust its internal diameter (calibre) to increase or decrease both the amount and the pressure of blood flowing through it. The third and inner layer is in two parts: a lining which is in contact with the circulating blood, and an elastic layer between the lining and the muscular, middle layer of the artery.

Arteries vary in size considerably – the aorta and the pulmonary artery are quite large as they leave the heart but gradually branch off into smaller and smaller arteries. When arteries become very small they are called arterioles. Arterioles link up with the capillaries, the smallest form of conduit, to supply blood to all the body tissues.

THE CAPILLARIES

Capillaries are tiny channels whose walls are only one cell thick and loosely formed to allow cells to pass through them. Capillaries form a very dense network throughout the body to ensure that all the body tissues are supplied with blood. As the blood passes through the capillary walls, it transfers oxygen and nutrients to the tissue cells and collects waste material and carbon dioxide from them. Because the capillary walls are permeable, this transfer is able to take place instantly without the flow of blood being impaired. The permeable nature of the capillaries also accounts for the speed with which white blood cells accumulate at the site of a wound or infection.

Once the blood cells have exchanged oxygen and nutrients for waste products, they must move away from the tissues in order to excrete that waste. The flow of blood continues, but now it is flowing *towards* the heart. To accomplish this return circulation, the capillaries gradually join up to form venules (small veins) and these in turn join and thicken to become veins.

THE VEINS
Veins are, externally, slightly smaller than arteries but with a larger interior diameter. Their walls are constructed of the same three layers of tissue described for arteries except that each layer is much thinner because the pressure of blood within a vein is much less than the pressure within an artery. Veins are also less elastic than arteries, so there are valves within some veins to prevent the back-flow of blood. These two factors, reduced pressure and reduced elasticity, mean that the veins in your body function at their best when your over all muscle tone is good. Your muscles support the veins and help to prevent collapse of the vein or back-flow of blood, as seen in varicose veins.

Veins always carry blood back to the heart.

THE SYSTEM AGAIN
Let's fit the various parts of the circulatory system together now, so that you can understand the marvelous cycle of events that is happening in your body every moment of your life.

Blood enters the top, right chamber of your heart through one of three veins, or openings. Once in this atrium, the thin muscle walls contract and the blood is pushed through a one-way valve into the right ventricle.

Almost immediately, the walls of the right ventricle contract powerfully and the blood is pushed through another valve into the pulmonary artery. The pulmonary artery divides almost immediately and channels the blood directly to your lungs. In the lungs, the arteries narrow into arterioles and these become a network of tiny capillaries. Once in the capillaries, the red blood cells exchange carbon dioxide, which is excreted as you exhale, for the oxygen present in your lungs. The haemoglobin

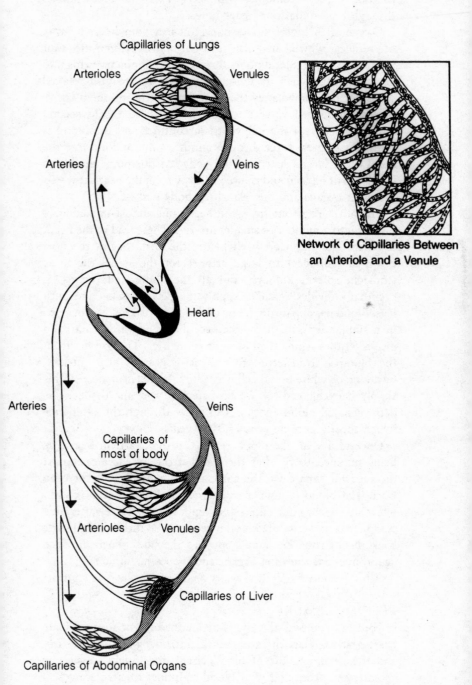

Capillaries of Lungs

Arterioles

Venules

Arteries

Veins

Network of Capillaries Between
an Arteriole and a Venule

Heart

Arteries

Veins

Capillaries of
most of body

Arterioles

Venules

Capillaries of Liver

Capillaries of Abdominal Organs

in your red cells combines with oxygen as your blood moves through the capillaries of your lungs.

Oxygen-rich blood moves back towards your heart by way of venules which, in turn, thicken and become the four pulmonary veins. Blood pours through the pulmonary veins into he left atrium when its muscle walls are in are in a relaxed state. Almost immediately the atrium contracts and the blood is pushed through a valve into he left ventricle. A split second later, the walls of the left ventricle contract and the blood is pushed with great force through another valve and out into the aorta – the largest artery in the body. At this point the blood is still full of oxygen and is moving away from the heart, towards the other organs and the rest of the body tissues.

The aorta rises out from the heart and almost immediately divides into a number of smaller arteries. These lead to the head, the arms and the heart itself before the aorta begins to curve down and divide into large arteries for the spine, the liver, stomach, spleen, kidneys, and all the abdominal organs. It eventually divides again to supply the pelvic organs and both legs. Blood passing through any one of these arteries is processed in a similar way to that described above: the artery narrows into arterioles which then become capillaries. The oxygen from the blood is transferred to the tissues, as is any nutrient, hormone or white blood cell according to the tissue needs. This supply is exchanged for waste materials from the tissues. The deoxygenated blood continues to move through the capillaries which shortly become venules, then veins.

Once in a vein, the blood returns to the heart. In fact, it is being pumped to re-enter the heart at one of three openings: the superior vena cava, the coronary sinus or the inferior vena cava. The blood is high in waste material and low in oxygen when it, once again, enters the right atrium. Here, after this complete round-trip, the blood is recirculated through the lungs, back through the heart and out into the body where it, once again, interacts with the organs and tissues it supplies.

BLOOD PRESSURE

In your body, blood pressure is maintained by the force of your heart beat, the elasticity and natural narrowing of your arteries, and the total amount of blood circulating. Such pressure is necessary in order that your blood continues to circulate.

The volume of blood in your body at any one time and the

Diagram of the Circulation

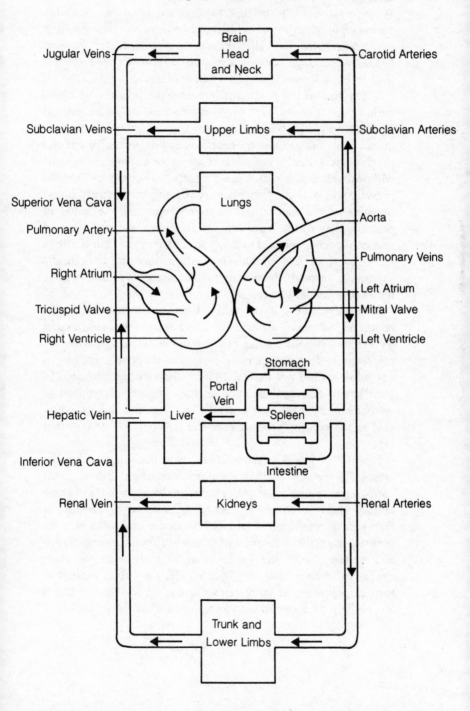

natural arrangement of arteries in an ever-narrowing network establishes a basic pressure within the walls of your arteries. When your heart is in that split-second state of relaxation between pumps (contraction of the chamber walls), this pressure may be measured. It is called diastole or diastolic blood pressure. Diastolic blood pressure in a healthy person is approximately 90 mm Hg (mercury rising to 90 millimetres in a glass tube).

When your heart pumps, it increases the pressure of blood within your arteries. This pressure may also be measured and is called systole or systolic blood pressure. Systole is subject to great changes depending on your age, health, physiological and psychological state. If you are exercising, for instance, your heart will probably pump with a greater force, so your systolic blood pressure will increase. Other factors affecting your systolic blood pressure are the internal size of your arteries and the degree of elasticity they retain. Your arteries naturally divide into smaller and smaller channels and in doing so contribute to your diastolic blood pressure. But should your arteries become unnaturally narrowed, through disease or loss of elasticity, your systolic blood pressure will increase to an unhealthy level.

In healthy adults, systolic blood pressure should be in the region of 100 plus your age. So, an adult aged 35 could expect a maximum systolic reading of 135 mm Hg. In old age, however, this formula does not apply as the maximum systolic reading in any adult should not exceed 145 to 150 mm Hg (although in poor health the readings may be much higher). Diastolic and systolic blood pressure are generally read together and are expressed as the systolic pressure over the diastolic, i.e. 135/90 mm Hg.

Pressure of blood in the veins is lower than that within the arteries. So much so that the veins are often distended, or varicose, in persons whose circulation is impaired for some reason. Usually, however, a sufficient amount of pressure is maintained from the flow of blood from the capillaries into the venules, from the pressure and support of surrounding organs and muscle tissue, and from the suction effect as the chest expands during inhalation. Additionally, the valves located at various points in the large veins prevent a back-flow of blood and so help to maintain blood pressure within the veins.

IN SICKNESS OR IN HEALTH

You can see that the cardiovascular system is a finely tuned blend of mechanical and chemical functions that work together to sustain your health. As with any finely tuned system, however, if one small aspect of the system is disrupted or unbalanced then the whole system falters and sickness is a short heart-beat away, though not always obviously so. You have read, in brief, how the cardiovascular system should function. The next chapter describes how it might function when one or more of its features are altered through disorder or disease.

CHAPTER THREE
When Something Goes Wrong

The great majority of us are born with a healthy heart and enjoy continued cardiovascular health throughout childhood. Then, depending on environment, diet, lifestyle and a host of related factors, approximately half of us begin to develop some form of cardiovascular disease. In fact, many of us begin this development in early childhood. So, for a shocking number of people, disease slowly and gradually erodes their health, often without them being in the slightest bit aware that this is occurring. Why?

The answer is two-fold. In the first place, the symptoms of disease and the disease process are often not apparent to us. In the second place, we do not do all that we can to test whether or not cardiovascular disease is developing. Two tests in particular – a test to measure blood pressure and another to measure cholesterol levels in the blood – are readily available in the United Kingdom and could be crucial to the arrest and reversal of many cases of cardiovascular disease. Both tests are simple and quick to perform, yet neither of these tests is used widely enough. In fact, I would venture that fewer than one-quarter of adults know their blood pressure and that only a very tiny number of people know the level of cholesterol in their blood.

CURING IGNORANCE
Disease rises out of weakness or vulnerability which is either inherited or acquired. In this book, we will focus on acquired diseases of the cardiovascular system, rather than inherited ones. Weakness within the cardiovascular system is acquired through neglect, ignorance or as a result of another disease. Therefore, in order to minimise the likelihood of becoming ill it is necesssary to actively strengthen your body – especially your cardiovascular system – and to reverse the conditions of neglect and ignorance.

Health is maintained and enhanced when you attend to the

relationships between various parts of your body, between varius systems in your body, between your body, your attitude and your lifestyle. When you do not attend to these relationships, the network of good health gradually weakens and breaks apart until you suffer disorder or disease.

The problem is, few of us have a clear understanding of what our body does and what it needs to remain well. Unfortunately, such ignorance often creates fear and inaction leading you to neglect yourself. Obviously, the more you learn about your body, the better able you will be to care for it. We looked at the healthy cardiovascular system in chapter Two, now let's learn how the cardiovascular system functions when diseased.

TWIN TROUBLES

For many of us, the first we know of trouble with our health, or that of someone close to us, is when something drastic happens. When a colleague has an angina attack, or a relative has a stroke or heart attack, we often react with amazement: it all seems so sudden! Yet there are two diseases of the cardiovascular system which develop gradually and quietly over the years and eventually cause the events which seem so sudden and drastic to us.

These diseases are hypertension (high blood pressure) and atherosclerosis (hardening and narrowing of the arteries). These diseases may exist by themselves within a person, or they may develop together, one causing weakness that enables the other to become established.

Both diseases may now be 'discovered' during their early stages using two very simple tests. The test for high blood pressure is non-invasive, painless and very quick. The test for atherosclerosis is based on an assumption: that if the serum cholesterol count in a blood sample is above an agreed figure, then the person is almost certain to have build up of atheroma in their arteries. This test requires that a blood sample is taken (from the tip of the finger). Both tests are important in preventing unnecessary illness and death from these diseases. Here is a more detailed description of hypertension and atherosclerosis, followed by the other cardiovascular diseases that can result from them.

HIGH BLOOD PRESSURE

Without sufficient pressure your blood would not circulate properly and you would suffer dizziness, fainting or even death. Therefore, you need a blood pressure high enough to ensure proper circulation of the blood, but low enough to avoid damaging the heart and arteries. Most doctors and insurance companies consider that a blood pressure reading of approximately 140/90 mm Hg is the upper limit to their 'normal' assessment for adults under the age of sixty-five. Any higher than that reading is placed within their 'high blood pressure' assessment.

Blood pressure is measured using an instrument with an impossible name of the sphygmomanometer! It consists of an inflatable bag which is wrapped round your arm. The inside of this bag is connected by a rubber tube to a mercury filled pressure gauge. When the bag is inflated to the same degree of pressure as that of the blood within your artieres, the flow of blood is briefly interrupted. By listening through a stethoscope or by feeling the pulse it is possible to detect when this interruption occurs. At this pont the height of mercury within the gauge is noted: this is your systolic blood pressure, the first number in your reading. Now the bag is slowly deflated and, as the bag deflates, the mercury drops. To obtain the diastolic blood pressure, it is necessary to listen to the pulse as the bag deflates and the mercury drops. Your diastolic pressure is recorded as the point on the mercury gauge when you can no longer hear the pulse. Now you have both figures in your reading.

Use this list as a general guideline to determine what your own blood pressure should measure:

- the diastolic reading for a healthy adult should remain below 90 mm Hg
- the systolic reading should not drop below 100 mm Hg in healthy adults. If it does, it is likely that the person requires medical attention
- the systolic reading should approximate 100 plus the age of the adult, but not to exceed 140, if possible. (Age-induced rise in systolic pressure slows in those over sixty.) For instance:

Normal Systolic Blood Pressure	mm HG
age 20–30	100–120
age 30–60	120–140
over age 60	140–150

- women may have a systolic pressure that reads 10–20 mm

Hg less than healthy adult men at the same age. This is still considered normal.

- blood pressure readings may reach very high figures in both systolic and diastolic measurements (e.g. 190/110 mm Hg) but these are not considered at all healthy.

It is a good idea to have your blood pressure measured at least once each year because, as you will learn shortly, your blood pressure may climb higher than is healthy for you without any obvious symptoms. If you regularly check your blood pressure hoever, you can, if necessary, take early preventative action to keep it within healthy limits.

HIGH READINGS: NATURAL OR UNNATURAL?

There are many occasions when it is natural for your blood pressure to soar. If you have your blood pressure checked after you have just run for your bus, you are undoubtedly going to register a blood pressure that is higher than usual for you.

Although it is normal and natural for your blood pressure to vary according to circumstances, or even the time of day, when your blood pressure is persistently, or chronically, high you must consider it a problem. Chronic high blood pressure is called hypertension and the person who suffers it is called hypertensive. The simplest way of describing the arteries of a hyptertensive person is 'constricted'. That is, the arteries and arterioles are narrower and less flexible than in a healthy person. This means that the blood must push through them at greater force – a higher pressure – in order to circulate. And in order to provide that higher pressure, the heart must pump harder all of the time.

Your arterioles and arteries may become constricted temporarily, as happens in stress or fear, when signals sent through the nervous system cause your muscles and arteries to contract in tension. This sort of situation causes a corresponding, temporary rise in blood pressure. On the other hand, arterial constriction – and therefore high blood pressure – may become chronic due to physical or chemical changes in the profile of the artery and its surrounding tissues.

Physical changes include:

- a hardening and thickening of the artery walls (see Athero-sclerosis below)
- obesity

35

- a gross loss of tone in the muscles surrounding the artery such as occurs through lack of exercise.

Chemical changes include:

- a loss of nutrients and oxygen to needy cells as happens in malnutrition or anemia
- the introduction of toxic substances that alter the functioning of healthy cells and arterial blood flow (query any drugs you are taking)
- eating too much salt
- eating animal fat
- smoking
- drinking in excess
- feeling stressful
- taking the contraceptive pill.

Each of these factors will be discussed in greater detail in chapter four.

What are the symptoms?

Many people with high blood pressure don't know they have it until it is measured by their doctor, or until they have a heart attack or a stroke. Others, however, suffer from frequent headaches and chronic fatigue which leads them to have a check-up. In fact, the symptoms of hyptertension are rather non-specific and could as easily be caused by something other than high blood presure. This is why having your blood pressure measured once each year is such a good idea.

But if hypertension is so difficult to spot, why is it so important? The answer lies with those constricted arterioles. In healthy arteries, the flexible nature provided by muscle and elastic tissues enables the artery to respond to changes in blood pressure by contracting or relaxing somewhat. In constricted arteries this flexibility is inhibited and the result is that blood circulating under high pressure damages the inner lining of the artery. Then, a vicious cycle of constriction, inflexibility and damage is begun and, unless the blood pressure is reduced, this damaging cycle is sustained until a more drastic manifestation of the disorder is experienced – such as a heart attack or stroke.

How the disease develops

When blood is circulated at higher than normal pressure through your arteries it places too much stress on your arteries. Two things happen to damage the arteries. First, the muscle and elastic fibres in the middle layer of the artery extend in order to accommodate the higher pressure. This is a normal reaction, as mentioned earlier; however, if the period of extension is sustained for a prolonged length of time – as it would in chronic hypertension – the artery loses its elasticity and flexibility. Instead, the artery becomes 'hardened'. Now the second stage of damage has an opportunity to occur. When the artery loses its flexibility it is less able to adjust to fluctuations in blood pressure. So when blood pressure rises, or remains very high, the lining of the artery begins to erode or become chafed. These damaging stages mark the onset of atherosclerosis.

ARTERIOSCLEROSIS AND ATHEROSCLEROSIS

Arteriosclerosis is the name given to three distinct disease processes which cause a gradual and significant hardening and narrowing of the arteries. In one form, the arteries are hardened by a gradual deposition of calcium in the middle, muscle layer of the artery walls. In a second form, the small arteries, arterioles, become hardened and thick. And in the third, most familiar, form the large and medium sized arteries acquire a build-up of cholesterol, fats, blood cells and calcium on their inner layers. This last form is called atherosclerosis.

It is thought that hypertension may be one cause or contributing factor in the development of atherosclerosis. Certainly, once either disease is apparent, the other is usually not long in manifesting itself. Whichever disease comes first, the resulting loss of arterial flexibility increases the likelihood of further damage being done to the lining of the arteries and eventually to the heart itself. Here is the process described.

How the disease develops

When the artery lining is weakened or damaged, muscle tissues from the middle layer of the artery wall multiply and grow into the artery. Then fat molecules already in the blood begin to collect at the site of the damage. Blood normally carries fat molecules so that it may transfer them to body tissues. But when the concentration of fat in the blood is too high or when the artery wall is damaged, these molecules begin to form into plaques which adhere to the artery walls. A build up of fat at specific places along the lining of an already weak and damaged artery increases the stress placed on the artery and it bleeds into the fatty deposits. The white cells in the blood try to fight off bacteria and inflammation while the red cells combine with the platelets in the blood and begin a clotting process. This

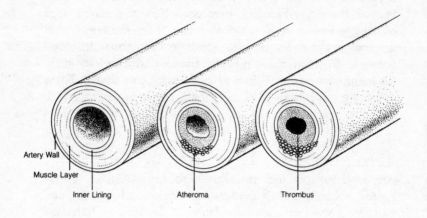

Artery Wall
Muscle Layer
Inner Lining   Atheroma   Thrombus

combination of fatty deposit and clotting blood is called *atheroma*.

The development of atheroma is gradual, often taking place over decades without the victim being aware of it. Atheroma can be a cause of death, however. When a deposit eventually blocks an artery, the blood flow is stopped and, with it, the supply of oxygen to tissue cells. This causes death to the deprived tissues and, if occurring in the heart muscle, a heart attack follows (see *heart attack* below).

But the disease process has further to go. Once the build-up of fat and blood begins, calcium deposits begin to harden the atheroma – especially in people entering late middle age. As the atheroma hardens and becomes brittle, it too can break from the artery wall and float away in the blood where, further along, it may block the artery. This form of blockage is called an embolism. The place in your artery where the brittle atheroma broke away is left raw and bleeding and a blood clot soon forms – called a thrombus. That clot may either block the artery there and then, or it too may break away and block the artery further along.

In both embolism and thrombosis there is further damage done to the artery and, more importantly, both create an obstruction of the blood flow through the artery. Loss of blood flow means loss of essential oxygen and nutrients, therefore an obstruction such as this usually means subsequent death of the affected tissue. If the obstruction occurs in or near the heart, a heart attack occurs. If in the brain, a stroke occurs. If this obstruction occurs in the eye, a degree of blindness may ensue and if in the extremities, death of tissue may cause gangrene and require amputation of the affected part.

What causes atherosclerosis?

It now seems likely that diet and lifestyle *combined* can be the cause of atherosclerosis and, as a result, of handicap or death by heart attack or stroke. As we'll see later, a reversal of some diet and lifestyle patterns can therefore prevent or reduce the incidence of cardiovascular disease. Here are the major aspects of diet and lifestyle which are thought to contribute to the development of atherosclerosis:

Aspects of diet:

- fat, particularly satured fat and cholesterol (in meat and dairy products)
- low fibre intake

Aspects of lifestyle:

- stress.
- lack of exercise
- smoking
- obesity

TREBLE TROUBLE

Hypertension and atherosclerosis are cardiovascular diseases which may appear alone or together, with or without obvious symptoms, in both men and women. Both diseases may cause discomfort, handicap and death and both contribute to the ischemic (deficiency in blood) forms of cardiovascular disease. In addition, and only briefly discussed here, there is a strong relationship between hypertension, atherosclerosis and cerebrovascular accident – also known as stroke.

There are two basic types of stroke. The first is an aneurysm or hemorrhage. This is the rupture of a blood vessel, such as an arteriole or capillary, that has been weakned by consistently high blood pressure. The second type is an obstruction of a blood vessel by atheroma (embolism) or by a blood clot

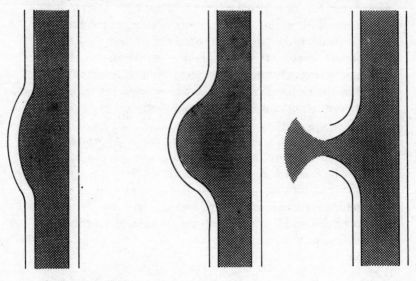

(thrombus). Both types of stroke have the result of killing nerve cells in the brain, leaving the area of body controlled by those nerve cells unable to function. Typically a stroke victim may suffer paralysis, impaired speech, loss of memory, confusion, or death. Those who experience a mild stroke have a chance of good recovery through the many therapeutic methods currently employed, such as physiotherapy, speech therapy and correction of diet and lifestyle habits.

An incredible eighty percent of stroke victims have a history of high blood pressure, half have cardiovascular disease and about one in ten victims have had a previous 'incident', either cardio- or cerebrovascular in nature. Many suffer from diabetes. The factors in diet and lifestyle already mentioned in terms of hypertension and atherosclerosis appear guilty also of contributing to the onset of a stroke.

ISCHEMIC HEART DISEASE
During exercise, stress, or when you are subject to the cold your heart needs to pump harder to maintain a sufficient supply of blood to your tissues. In a healthy person this occurs without any problem, though you may become slightly flushed or breath-

less. However, when the arteries and arterioles are constricted, as in atherosclerosis, hypertension or through nervous reaction, your heart must work even harder to supply adequate blood to your body tissues. Sometimes it doesn't succeed.

'Ischemic' means an insufficient supply of blood. Therefore ischemic heart disease is an insufficient supply of blood to the myocardium, or heart muscle. There are three forms of this disease, angina pectoris, myocardial infarction and sudden death.

ANGINA PECTORIS

In angina pectoris the heart itself becomes deprived of the blood needed to supply its own muscle tissues. This may be due to atheroma which narrows the coronary arteries, or it may occur when the arteires are constricted by nervous reaction, from stress, or the cold. In either case, the result is a strong, distinctive pain in the region of the heart. This pain is often described as 'vice-like, aching, tight, heavy or dull and is usually felt in the chest. In some angina sufferers, the pain may radiate to the neck, arms (especially the left arm) or even the back.

The pain of angina pectoris is usually eased with rest (unlike a heart attack, where the pain is prolonged and does *not* disappear with rest). Additionally, the underlying cause of angina may be treated in several ways so that the symptoms are minimized or disappear altogether. Drug treatment is an obvious means of affecting the course of angina pectoris, which can disable or cause death if left to progress. However, improving one's level of fitness and finding ways of coping with all forms of stress in everyday life are measures that may be taken immediately to prevent or relieve the threat of angina. Diet and lifestyle are, once gain, important factors in both the cause and the prevention of angina pectoris.

MYOCARDIAL INFARCTION

The myocardium is the muscular wall of the heart and, like all muscle tissue, it is supplied with oxygenated blood which circulates through the coronary arteries and may become obstructed in the same way as other arteries in the body. When obstruction is only partial some blood gets through and the heart only suffers when it is challenged – as with angina pectoris.

When the obstruction is total, however, the area of myocar-

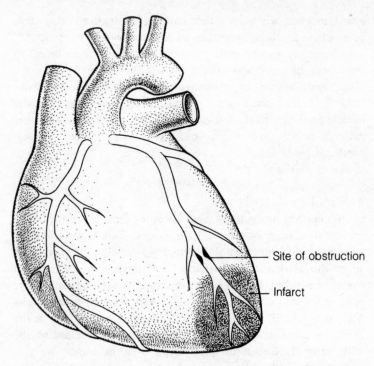

Site of obstruction

Infarct

dium that is completely deprived of blood dies. This area of dead tissue is called an infarct. The process of obstruction, pain and death of tissue is called a myocardial infarction – or heart attack. Heart attacks may be caused by obstruction of the coronary arteries due to atherosclerosis, embolism or a blood clot (thrombus). In some cases, atheroma and coronary thrombosis are both present and together contribute to the heart attack.

The area of myocardium affected by the obstruction stops contracting, or pumping, when it is deprived of blood and that area of tissue dies shortly after, usually within hours. This period of time is very painful for the victim. If the victim survives the heart attack, the myocardium in the region of the obstruction becomes scar tissue. This is dead tissue which the body cannot replace. If the obstructed artery supplied a small area of myocardium, then the infarct, or scar, will be relatively small also. If, however, a larger coronary artery is obstructed the infarct will be larger. A large infarct is more likely to cause a loss of heart rhythm and, in some people, the sudden loss of heart rhythm due to infarct causes immediate death. In other victims the area of muscle tissue affected is so small that no symptoms are felt

– this is called 'silent infarct'. A number of 'silent infarcts' may occur before a major heart attack is experienced.

During a heart attack the victim suffers from persistent pains similar to those described for angina. That is, vice-like, tight, crushing pains that radiate to the neck, jaw, arms and sometimes the back. These pains may last for hours or even days and do *not* disappear with rest or altering position. In addition, the victim may have symptoms such as profuse sweating, vomiting, nausea, feelings of cold and a sense of doom. In the event of any of these symptoms appearing in someone close to you *hospital treatment must be sought immediately* to prevent death.

SUDDEN DEATH

Sudden death is often the first sign of any cardiovascular disease. Although it may be caused by injury, it is more often due to a combination of atherosclerosis and ischemia which acts swiftly and profoundly on the victim. Such people are often said to die 'instantly'. There is no treatment for this form of heart attack and no way of predicting it. The causes, which are in common with those of all other forms of cardiovascular disease, provide the only insight as to how it may be prevented.

For the majority of heart attack victims, their attack was the first they knew of any cardiovascular problems. Only one in every four or five victims were known to have had symptoms of hypertension or angina prior to their heart attack. Yet, undoubtedly, hypertension and its companion, atherosclerosis, are the basic disorders underlying myocardial infarction. Therefore, it is important that we consider how to prevent or minimize these conditions if we wish to reduce the incidence of stroke, angina pectoris, heart attack, and sudden death. The following two chapters deal with aspects of lifestyle and diet that contribute to cardiovascular disease. However, where there's a cause, there is a cure and diet and lifestyle may be altered to provide protection from the epidemic of cardiovascular disease.

CHAPTER FOUR
Lifestyle Culprits & Cures

Lifestyle is a blend of many things: attitude, environment, wealth, activity, even hopes and dreams. It is a combination of both vague and definite factors in our lives which in some way affect its outcome. Lifestyle can cause or contribute to cardiovascular disease, yet it can become part of the cardiovascular 'cure' as well. The recommendations made here are intended to help you prevent cardiovascular disease or to minimise its effects if you have already developed it. After all, prevention is the most powerful and effective medicine in the world, one which you may be able to give to those you love.

ALCOHOL

An occasional 'drink' may be a pleasant and social experience, but in large quantities it can cause liver disorders, heart and circulatory disease as well as gross mood and personality changes. Alcohol is also responsible for many cases of obesity and it has the effect of complicating, when taken in excess, almost every illness or disorder from which you may suffer. A fair amount of controversy surrounds the question of whether or not alcohol can actually cause cardiovascular disease. Certainly there are some very heavy drinkers who suffer from heart disease *because* they drink, but they are rare; moderate drinkers and those who drink no alcohol are the focus of this controversy.

Those who favour abstinence (teetotal) from drinking alcohol point out that alcohol is high in calories and therefore can contribute greatly to obesity, which is known to cause high blood pressure. And, as you know, high blood pressure can lead to other forms of cardiovascular disease. In addition, drinking alcohol is often associated with smoking which also contributes to hypertension and atherosclerosis.

The other point of view suggests that 'teetotallers' are actually at greater risk of cardiovascular disease than their alcohol drinking peers. The reasons why this is argued are derived from comparison between teetotallers and moderate drinkers where the moderate drinkers either did not seem to suffer any greater risk of cardiovascular disease, or actually suffered less from it than those who did not drink. These are some of the reasons put forward to support the case for moderate drinking:

- There doesn't appear to be evidence that alcohol by itself and in moderate amounts is harmful to most people's health
- moderate amounts may help to reduce feelings of stress and anxiety – both known to contribute to cardiovascular disease
- alcohol does dilate, or open, the blood vessels and so may ease somewhat the work load on the heart
- alcohol is usually drunk in a social context. This social environment may further reduce levels of stress and increase one's sense of belonging, a factor recognized as supporting overall good health

Both sides of the discussion have clear and sensible points to make and, certainly, both groups agree that excessive drinking is not good for any aspect of health on any level. So the choice is yours. If you decide to drink, however, moderation is crucial if you wish to preserve your health. What is moderation? The Greater London Alcohol Avisory Service (GLAAS) suggests that:

- women cosume *no more* than two to three units of alcohol, two to three times in a week
- men consume *no more* than four to six units of alcohol, two to three times in a week
- all drinkers have three or four drink-free days in each week
- all drinks are consumed slowly: one unit per hour, one unit at a time, preferably accompanied by food.
  One unit of alcohol equals:
  = one-half pint of beer
  = one measure of spirit
  = one glass of wine
  = 1 glass of sherry, vermouth or aperitif

A final caution: I strongly advise against heavy or immoderate drinking. Heavy drinking is *definitely* damaging to the heart, liver, stomach and brain. It raises blood pressure, increases weight and alters the level of cholesterol in the blood.

OBESITY

One-third of women and nearly 40% of men in the United Kingdom are considered by Department of Health and Social Security surveys to be very overweight. That means that approximately nine million women and over ten and a half million men treble their risk of developing diabetes, double their risk of having a high level of cholesterol in their blood, and suffer from hypertension. Obese people are nearly six times more likely to suffer from hypertension than un-obese people. And that is not to mention the social stigma attached to obesity which leaves people feeling ugly, guilty, embarrassed and generally less than socially acceptable.

This is an alarming number of people – and these figures do not include children. Currently, between 50/80% of British children are considered overweight and underactive – in fact, the obese adults of the future. Yet, most cases of obesity are not genetically caused and, as such, are within our control to change.

Let me first explain the difference between obesity and being overweight. Obesity means that you are between ten and twenty per cent over your ideal weight (see charts below). Being overweight means that you weigh up to ten percent more than is ideal for you. As with any issue that is potentially a problem, it is best to know the facts, and to learn the truth about your weight. For this reason, have a look at the charts which follow. They are drawn from the figures compiled by the Metropolitan Life Insurance Company of New York and give the upper and lower limits to weight for each category of height, frame and gender. If you are near to your upper weight limit, or if you are obviously over that limit, then read on about the steps you can take to reduce.

Obese people are prone to high blood pressure, though precisely why this should be so is not clear. Certainly an uncontrolled diet full of fats, salt and sugar would create high blood pressure and it is possible that many or most obese people eat in this way. But obesity also puts excess strain on the heart because blood must circulate to fatty tissue as well as, for instance, the organs and muscle tissue. With more tissue to support, the heart must pump harder in order to achieve proper circulation. Of course, your heart would much rather pump more slowly and easily to a less bulky body.

Obesity must be conquered if you wish to minimize your risk of suffering from cardiovascular disease. Easier said than done, however! Many people learn to be obese as children, others

Desirable Weights for Men and Women Aged 25 and Over

MEN: wearing indoor clothing and shoes with one-inch heels

Height	Small Frame lb	Medium Frame lb	Large Frame lb
5'2"	112–120	118–129	126–141
5'3"	115–123	121–133	129–144
5'4"	118–126	124–136	132–148
5'5"	121–129	127–139	135–152
5'6"	124–133	130–143	138–156
5'7"	128–137	134–147	142–161
5'8"	132–141	138–152	147–166
5'9"	136–145	142–156	151–170
5'10"	140–150	146–160	155–174
5'11"	144–154	150–165	159–179
6'0"	148–158	154–170	164–184
6'1"	152–162	158–175	168–189
6'2"	156–167	162–180	173–194
6'3"	160–171	167–185	178–199
6'4"	164–175	172–190	182–204

WOMEN: wearing indoor clothing and shoes with two-inch heels

Height	Small Frame lb	Medium Frame lb	Large Frame lb
4'10"	92–98	96–107	104–119
4'11"	94–101	98–110	106–122
5'0"	96–104	101–113	109–125
5'1"	99–107	104–116	112–128
5'2"	102–110	107–119	115–131
5'3"	105–113	110–122	118–134
5'4"	108–116	113–116	121–138
5'5"	111–119	116–130	125–142
5'6"	114–123	120–135	129–146
5'7"	118–127	124–139	133–150
5'8"	122–131	128–143	137–154
5'9"	126–135	132–147	141–158
5'10"	130–140	136–151	145–163
5'11"	134–144	140–155	149–168
6'0"	138–148	144–159	153–173

NOTE: for each year under 25, women between the ages of 18 and 24 should subtract one pound from the upper limit of their 'category'. Weight measured in the nude may be two to five pounds less than that measured in indoor clothing.

gradually gain weight as they become adult and, through their middle years, continue to put on a pound here and there. Some obese people seem to eat anything that is put in front of them, others eat less than their slim friends and relations. The problem, however it arose is still excess weight.

Here is a list of ten tips to help you reduce your weight at the same time as you care for your cardiovascular system. The diet and recipes included in this book will also help you to lose weight, although they are designed specifically with your heart and arteries in mind. For more information on weight reduction, see the Appendix at the end of this book.

- Eat at least three times per day – current opinion is that starving yourself in order to lose weight will mean the weight comes on more easily later. Apparently your metabolism alters so that you actually store fat cells better and in greater quantity if your body thinks there is a famine! It is *what* you eat that will make the difference.
- When you eat, eat slowly, chew well and try not to do anything apart from eat at that time. You'll find that you will feel more satisifed with your meal if it is eaten in this way.
- Cut down on foods such as red meat, poultry, fish, eggs, milk products and – sorry – avocados! These are very obviously fatty foods and they are probably contributing a great deal to your being overweight.
- Cut your consumption of the remaining fats in half. For instance, if you normally sauté the onions and mushrooms in two tablespoons of oil, saute them in one tablespoon instead. Similarly with your consumption of peanut butter, margarine, tahini and any other fats you use regularly. After one month, cut your consumption of these in half again.
- Eat at least one pound of any fresh, raw fruit and one pound of any fresh, raw vegetable each day (or a combination of fruit and vegetables).
- 60–70% of your food should be from the complex carbo-hydrate group which includes whole grains, fruits, vegetables, beans, pulses, nuts and seeds. Prepare these without oils, salt or sugar.
- Stop taking sugar. Leave it out of your hot drinks and avoid eating it in cakes, cereals, jams and spreads.
- Double the amount of exercise you do. See the *Exercise* entry below for more details. And no skimping!

- Weigh yourself weekly – no more, no less. Keep a record of your weight as it changes and reward yourself for each weight loss you achieve. Just make sure the reward isn't food!
- Keep a notebook in which you write down how you behave around food. This will make you more aware of behaviour that might contribute to your obesity. Once you become aware in this way, you have more power to change and control your behaviour.

For instance, do you notice that you always finish off whatever is left of a meal? Well, it's not doing *you* much good and, chances are, there are other ways of stopping it going to waste. Why not freeze it or refrigerate it for use in a lunch box the next day? It may be that a great deal of your weight problem is behavioural and, that by changing the way you do some things, you could really begin to conquer your obesity.

If you are a parent, altering your behaviour will benefit your children. If they see that you are obese, they may well learn how to be obese themselves, just by watching how you prepare and eat your food.

SMOKING

If you smoke cigarettes, you run twice the risk of having a heart attack compared to a non-smoker. If you have high blood pressure, high levels of cholesterol in your blood and you smoke, you run eight times the risk of having a fatal heart attack. In fact, eight out of ten deaths from cardiovascular disease in young men are thought to be caused by smoking.

Smoking seems to compound the unhealthy effects of obesity, lack of exercise, high blood pressure and high levels of cholesterol so that your total risk from cardiovascular disease is increased. In women, smoking increases the dangerous side effects of the contraceptive pill and complicates arterial problems in the legs. And there is no doubt that smoking causes cardiovascular disease.

We have learned how the red blood cells contain a substance, called haemoglobin, which combines with oxygen and transports it to needy tissue cells. Yet, in chronic smokers the oxygen-carrying capacity of red blood cells can be reduced by fifteen per cent. The reason is that cigarette smoke contains carbon monoxide and the haemoglobin in your red blood cells combines more easily with this poisonous gas than it does with oxygen, and forms a compound called carboxy-haemoglobin.

Carboxy-haemoglobin increases the permeability, or openness, of the artery walls so that more fats are able to lodge there. The build-up of fats which results effectively narrows the arteries (atherosclerosis) and increases the risk of heart attack. When the supply of carbon monoxide is fairly sustained, as it would be in a regular smoker, this damaging compound is transported to the tissues in a consistent ratio of one to every six or seven cells containing oxygen. Which means that, when you smoke, atherosclerosis is being given the best possible circumstances in which to develop.

Remember that your body tissues need oxygen. During a shortage, in order to get the amount of oxygen necessary for your cells to survive, the heart pumps harder to move the blood more quickly through the arteries. If only five out of six red blood cells carry oxygen, your heart needs to work fifteen per cent harder than the heart of a non-smoker.

In summary, if you are a smoker, your blood is depleted in oxygen and contains a poison that causes your arteries to narrow; so your heart must work harder to get oxygen-carrying blood through to the cells that need it. Unfortunately, this is exactly the cycle of events necessary to create high blood pressure, atherosclerosis, stroke, heart attack. Before you claim 'oh, but I don't inhale', let me tell you about the other major poison in cigarette smoking that affects your cardiovascular system.

Nicotine, the addictive substance in tobacco that is probably the reason for your habit in the first place, stimulates your nerves in such a way that they constrict your blood vessels. One result is that your heart has to work *even harder* and faster in order to keep the blood circulating.

Put carbon monoxide and nicotine together and you have a lethal combination of substances that almost guarantee to set you on the path of cardiovascular doom and destruction.

- both substances cause constriction in the arteries
- both substances increase the work load of the heart
- both substances affect the blood in such a way that it clots more easily in the arteries.

It really doesn't make sense to carry on smoking, does it? Here are ten tips to help you quit:

- Make the decision to quit *yourself* and be really committed in your decision. In the end it is your personal choice and commitment that achieve success, not someone else's pressure or jibes.

- Plan how you are going to quit – what you will do when you feel tempted, how you will talk about it, and when you will start to stop. Planning makes the whole process more formal and more real.

- Remove all the cigarettes, lighters and ashtrays from your home and work place, thus eliminating obvious temptation.

- If possible, make your 'personal space', such as home and office, a no-smoking zone, for everyone, and spend much of your time in these places.

- Select seats in the no-smoking areas of trains, buses and restaurants to keep you away from temptation.

- Treat yourself to special meals that are outside of your routine eating pattern. Smoking is often an after-meal habit. Change the style of meal and you might change the habit.

- Reward yourself for each day passed without a cigarette. Many ex-smokers complain that they gained weight in the first weeks after quitting. Therefore, make sure you don't make food one of your rewards. Why not make going to the opera, cinemas or local yoga class your reward instead?

- Put the money you would have spent on cigarettes in a separate box or wallet and use it for something you have always wanted. You'll be amazed at how quickly it reaches treble figures.

- Use some sort of replacement activity for the first four to six weeks after quitting. Be creative and think up a five-minute experience that will help you achieve your goal. A quick game of solitaire, writing a postcard to a distant relative, or telephoning an understanding friend may be just the answer to these difficult moments.

- Support your decision and your new lifestyle by making one or two other changes in your life as well. For instance, it's well known that your senses of taste and smell improve after you've quit smoking for a few months. Why not attend a wine tasting or cookery class and make full use of these 'new' senses? Or join a sports team or exercise class to make use of your 'new' lungs.

One final word of encouragement. When you do stop smoking, your risk of suffering a fatal heart attack willl begin to decline *immeidately*. And within five to ten years you will have the same level of risk as a life-long non-smoker. Good luck.

STRESS

Stress is a reaction. Stress causes your body to respond to a situation as though a solution must be found urgently. And however much you try to keep this reaction a solely mental one stress always has physical symptoms too. Here is what happens:

When you feel stressful, your adrenals make a hormone called adrenaline which prepares your body for urgent action. This physical response is ancient, an inheritance from our ancestors, and is often called the 'fight or flight' response. In other words, your body prepares for immediate hard work by producing a hormone that will trigger other important bodily responses.

Whenever you work hard, in fact, even when you anticipate having to work hard, our body requires more oxygen. During stress your body works hard and needs additional oxygen, so your heart starts to beat faster and harder, your blood pressure rises, your breathing becomes faster – all in order to help you either beat a fast retreat or beat the problem. You also begin to perspire: your body thinks you're going to run fast or fight fast and so it perspires to keep you cool during your efforts. Some people also experience a dry mouth: a clever physical trick to stop you from eating at a stressful moment. If you did eat, your body would have to divert blood and oxygen to your digestive tract and away from your brain and muscles. Not a good idea if you intend urgent thought or movement!

At the same time, your liver triggers the release of fats and sugars directly into your blood stream to give you instant energy. Among these fats is cholesterol. If your body does not use the extra fats and sugars, the fats are available to line the arteries – thus contributing to the development of atheroma – and the sugars affect blood sugar levels so that other body functions are altered. All of this may occur when the stressful situation is left unresolved, so continually experiencing unresolved stress can aggravate hypertension, atherosclerosis and cause oxygen deprivation leading to angina or heart attack. If a person already suffers from atherosclerosis or high blood pressure, the stressful response may be just enough to tip the balance and cause the heart to overwork, a clot to finally block an artery, then a stroke or heart attack.

This whole pattern of physical response is really an excellent means of ensuring self-preservation. But *only* if we are able to complete the cycle and use our brains and bodies to get us through the stressful situation. In many modern day situations this is no longer possible. Very few of us would have a real punch-up with the boss (fight response) and it is unlikely that we would run away from the boss either (flight response). Yet, our bodies prepare us for just such an event.

In some countries stress does not contribute to cardiovascular disease. This may be due to other factors — including diet, smoking, level of exercise — or simply to the way stress is felt and dealt with. Here in the West, however, stress is a significant part of our health problem. Though we may not notice it contributing to cardiovascular disease, we surely notice its other symptoms, including:

headache	indigestion
ulcers	poor appetite
muscular stiffness	eczema
asthma	hostility

Stress can create a vicious cycle of events leading to ill health and even death. Of course, a little stress is natural and for some people even enjoyable. Many people would rather do without it however and, for them, new and better methods of responding to situations are needed. Here are ten guiding tips on how to deal with stress:

Dealing with the cause of stress

- You must first pinpoint the person, situation, or whatever it is that seems to trigger the stressful response in you. Once you have found it, think of precisely what aspect of that person or situation creates the stress. You should think in this way while you are away from the stressful situation and make a clear note of what you have deduced.
- Is there an obvious solution? Run through the situation again, as though it were a film, and note any aspect of it that you think you might be able to change.
- You might find it useful to talk the problem and/or the proposed solution through with someone else. Another point of view is often very helpful in coping with a challenge.
- Organize your stress so that it doesn't all happen to you at once. You are no doubt very familiar with the events, people and situations in your life that you find stressful. So take

control! Make sure that you don't allow more than one or two of these 'regulars' from happening on any one day.

- Try to change the way you react to the stress in your life. It is possible that your reaction to a situation is entirely responsible for the stress you are suffering. Here are a few means of altering your response and, in doing so, countering the effects of stress on your health.

Dealing with the effects of stress

- Relaxation is the opposite of tension. When you are stressful, your muscles tense, your breathing becomes tighter and more shallow, and your circulation becomes impaired. In order to counter stress or, better still, beat it before it gets a firm grip, you must attempt to trigger a relaxation response instead of a stress response. You can do this in a split second by telling yourself 'step back, turn around, start again'. This gives you a brief reprieve while you reverse the pattern of tension and stress.

'Step back' means that you mentally step away from the situation. This is a way of creating more inner space and time in which you can think clearly.

'Turn around' means that you mentally do a slow turn around of your reaction. In other words, you reverse it: where your muscles are tense, let them lose tension, where your breath is short and tight, take a deep breath. All of this can happen in a matter of two or three seconds!

Finally, 'start again' means that you mentally step forward and encounter the situation once more. But this time with a fresh, more relaxed response. Remember, every situation is yours to handle however you please. If you truly realize this you will increase your sense of control and, therefore, decrease your level of stress in most situations.

Another sure way to relax is to take a nap! Researchers from the University of Athens, in Greece, studied people at risk from coronary heart disease and found that a thirty-minute nap in the afternoon could reduce their risk of heart attack by as much as 30%. Elsewhere, scientists are 'discovering' what many people have known for ages – that holding and stroking a warm, furry animal soothes your *human* cares away too. In fact, it is possible that this gentle, sharing activity actually slows the heart beat and lowers blood pressure. What more encouragement do you need?

- Breathing is immediately affected by your mood and, in particular, your level of stress. Your body's natural response to the stress trigger is to breathe more rapidly in order to supply oxygen to your now rapid circulation. If you need or want to be stressed, then let your breathing continue in this way. However, if you want to decrease or neutralize the stress you are feeling, take charge of your breathing. Here is the most basic breathing pattern for this purpose:
- take one long, deep breath in
- hold it for three seconds
- then let the breath out slowly and, if you like, noisily
- repeat this five to ten times – usually long enough to stop the stress reaction from developing fully.

You might consider practising new patterns of breathing so that you gain real awareness and control of your breath. See the Appendix for information on further reading or teaching organisations to contact.

- Exercise can be of the sort that combines movement, breathing patterns, relaxation and time for meditation or contemplation. The benefit you gain from a yoga type exercise often lasts for several days. See the entry below for more information on exercise.
- Laughter can de-fuse the most stressful situation within seconds. It might be that you really can't find anything funny in the immediate situation, but you can certainly undermine the detrimental effects of residual or long-term stress by making sure that you get regular laughter sessions.
- Change is one of the building-blocks of life and our ability to accept change and participate in it is responsible for our surival and much of all human achievement. Yet, many of us are frightened of change and do all that we can to avoid it. If you react to change in this way, it is almost certain that you become stressful when a possibility of change appears in your life. Try to avoid this by varying your routine and habits occasionally, meet new people and develop fresh interest.

EXERCISE
Obesity and lack of exercise are often comparison lifestyle habits – each ensuring that the other is maintained. However, obesity may be cured by persistant and regular exercise, and exercise becomes easier with every pound of excess weight that is lost.

Regular exercise benefits the cardiovascular system because it:

reduces stress
reduces depression, agression and hostility
reduces blood pressure
reduces levels of fat in the blood (by using it for energy)
tones all muscle tissue – including heart muscle
keeps the arteries flexible
improves circulation and heart rate

Beneficial types of exercise are those that require:

the muscles to both stretch and contract
the joints to move
the brain to deal with co-ordination
the lungs to open for deep breathing
the heart to pump strongly and regulary

Static exercise such as bodybuilding is not useful to improve the health of your heart, neither is sport or exercise that you do not enjoy. Instead, pleasureable exercise such as dancing, swimming, yoga, walking, keep fit and many games are beneficial, and should be performed a minimum of three times each week for 20–30 minutes per session. At this rate, your overall fitness will improve, you will develop a sense of well-being and your heart will pump more slowly and efficiently when you are not exercising.

Ideally, exercise should become an integral part of your life, where you feel that something important is missing when you do *not* exercise. For this reason alone, it is best that the exercise you select is pleasureable. There is nothing to stop you from trying variety in your exercise either. You may cycle to and from the shops, walk your dog daily, go to keep fit once each week and still have the time and energy for one or two other exercise opportunities like dancing or swimming.

CONTRACEPTIVE PILL

Since the contraceptive pill for women became available, its effects on other aspects of women's health has been studied. Among the findings of these studies is a noticeable rise in blood pressure among some women using the pill. Therefore, if you use this method of contraception, you should have your blood pressure checked regularly (yearly). In addition, you should be doubly certain that you avoid smoking and becoming over-weight. It is possible that the risk of developing high blood pressure as a result of taking the contraceptive pill is higher in those women over the age of thirty-five.

The contraceptive pill is being continually altered in its strength and precise formulation and it is therefore likely that a change in the type of pill used will change the level of risk. It is also possible that new developments will completely or significantly reduce the risk of developing high blood pressure. Discuss any queries you might have regarding the pill you take with your doctor.

QUITE SIMPLY
Your health can be improved and cardiovascular disease prevented by following this three-point lifestyle plan:

1) Stop smoking
2) Control your weight, level of stress and alcohol intake
3) Take regular exercise

CHAPTER FIVE

Culinary Culprits & Cures

The dietary habits which you and most other people have grown up with are responsible, at least in part, for causing the epidemic scale of cardiovascular disease currently suffered here in the United Kingdom. The high-fat, high-sodium, low-fibre diet enjoyed since the war has become habitual to the majority of the population to the extent that it is called 'average' and 'traditional'. These words have a powerful effect – they imply safety, security, social acceptance – and many of us use them to stop ourselves thinking deeply or intelligently about what we eat and why we eat it.

Eating is *the* habit of a lifetime. What you eat, how you select and prepare your food, your attitude towards it – eating habits are something most of us learn from others, our parents for instance, and then continue to practice, as though they were our own, for the rest of our lives.

The result of a non-thinking state is an inertia which is not only detrimental to your health but is also precisely what some groups of people wish to encourage. The government, the medical profession and the food industry convey the message 'don't think and don't change'. How do they do this?

- by consistently supporting the current 'average' or 'traditional' diet through their unwillingness to encourage change
- by consistently doubting and undermining the medical and scientific facts and concerns which highlight the dangers of the diet they are supporting
- by consistently providing economic incentives for you and I to follow this 'average' diet and, in doing so, eat ourselves into an early grave.

You .can guess what I am about to ask you: please start thinking.

Certain aspects of diet are *known* to contribute to cardio-vascular disease and they are discussed below. Keep an open mind and decide for yourself whether your habits and traditions place you in a high-risk situation. And if they do, apply the recommended changes to your own diet and *prevent cardiovascular disease* for yourself and those your love.

FAT

When is the last time someone told you that fat is a good thing? Well, fat is a good thing but only if it constitutes 15–25% of your total body weight (for male and female, respectively). You need approximately this much fat in your body in order to be healthy because fat plays an important role in much of what your body does to keep alive and well.

For instance, fatty tissue surrounds your heart, liver and kidneys to protect and support them. And there is a thin layer of fat under the skin that helps you to maintain your body temperature by insulating you from outside extremes of cold and heat. When your food is digested, fat is transported through the blood stream to your body tissues, providing energy in a very accessible form. In addition, fat enters your blood stream carrying fat-soluble vitamins such as A, D and E which are essential to the health of all your body tissues and functions. That's the good news. The bad news is that it is easy to consume too much fat and that some of his fat has an especially unhealthy effect on the cardiovascular system.

Too Much

Today in Britain, the average quantity of fat consumed by every person each day is 40% of their total calorie intake. Recent recommendations[1] state that your total fat consumption should be reduced from the current average to a *maximum* of 25–30% . They state further that a *maximum* of 10% of your total calorie intake (less than half of your fat intake) comprise saturated fats such as lard, butter, cheese and other animal fats. The remaining 15% (at least) should come from unsaturated fats, such as vegetable oils, with at least 2% of that amount from fats high in linoleic acid, such as safflower, soybean, and corn oils. (Linoleic acid is an essential fatty acid, part of vitamin F, and must be supplied in your diet.) **NOTE:** One gram of fat equals nine calories. Use this equation to compute your current fat/calorie intake. See chapter Six for your recommended daily intake of calories and fats.

[1] i.e. *World Health Organisation Expert Committee Report on the Prevention of Coronary Heart Disease, 1982: NACNE Report 1983: COMA Report 1984.*

These recommendations call for an urgent reduction in total fat intake because a high-fat diet, especially one high in saturated fats, places a great strain on your body. It causes obesity, slows digestion and the absorption of essential nutrients and can ultimately cause cardiovascular disease.

Saturated and Unsaturated Fats

There are two basic types of fat (also called fatty acids of lipids). *Saturated fat* is usually solid when at roomtemperature. It includes animal fats such as lard, dripping, butter and also the fats from the coconut and palm plants. It is also present in meat, milk and eggs, as well as small amounts in some vegetable foods. *Unsaturated fat* is usually liquid at room temperature and is derived from vegetables, nuts and seeds. Some unsaturated fats are corn oil, olive oil and safflower oil. Solid or semi-solid forms of unsaturated fats can be made through a process of hydrogenation, as in many of the vegetable margarines currently available on the market.

Among the unsaturated fatty acids, three are considered 'essential', that is, we are unable to produce them within our bodies and so must take them in our food. These fatty acids are called vitamin F when referred to all together, individually they are called linoleic, arachidonic and linolenic acids. They ensure healthy blood, nerves and arteries and contribute to the health of skin and the process of normal growth. They also play an important role in the management of cholesterol.

Saturated fats have an ability to thicken the blood and increase its tendency to clot. Saturated fats in the diet also increase the amount of cholesterol in your plasma; as you will read below, cholesterol is the fatty deposit which accumulates on the artery walls to cause atherosclerosis. Unsaturated fats, especially those high in linoleic acid, have the ability to thin the blood and decrease the likelihood of blood clots and fatty build-up on the artery walls. These fats can actually decrease the level of cholesterol in your blood.

To minimize the amount of fat you include in your diet, select only those fats which in some way enhance your health. For instance, olive oil and oils high in linoleic acid are beneficial to the transportation of fatty acids and fat-soluble vitamins. Used in small amounts, they provide the flavour and 'body' that is often desired in a meal. Allow yourself and your family four to six weeks to gradually reduce your total fat intake and, at the same time, convert that intake from saturated to unsaturated fats.

60

Fats to Avoid	Fats to Use
Lard	Olive Oil
Dripping	Safflower or Soya Oil
Butter	Low-fat Spread (Margarine)
Coconut Oil	Corn or Sunflower Oil
Palm Oil	Nut or Seed Oils such as Tahini & Peanut Butter

- Avoid using oils that are labelled simply 'vegetable oil' as these tend to be a blend of oils and are often high in saturated fat. Instead, spend a little more and buy a 'cold-pressed' oil such as olive, safflower or sunflower.
- If cooking with oil, use it only once and then discard it. Oil cooked more than once changes its chemical composition and loses its health giving effects.
- Margarine has as many calories as butter and can be as high in saturated fats! Look for a label that reads 'high in polyunsaturates' to ensure that these beneficial fatty acids are included in the margarine you buy. Low-fat spreads usually contain only half the calories of butter or margarine and are useful to reduce total fat consumption and help you lose weight. They are not, however, particularly high in polyunsurates.

Some foods have very large quantities of hidden saturated fat and these foods should be eaten in very limited quantities, avoided if possible.

Fatty Foods To Limit	Less- or Non-Fatty Substitutes
Meat	Beans and Pulses
Fish	Tempeh (Soya Bean Meat)
Fowl	Vegetable Protein Products
Milk	Skimmed, Semi-skimmed Milk or, best, Soya Milk
Cheese	Low-fat Cottage Cheese, Quark or, best, Tofu (Soya Curd)
Eggs	Egg Replacer

Cholesterol
Cholesterol is an essential ingredient for a healthy body. It is a fat-like substance naturally present virtually everywhere in the body: it circulates in the blood and is found in nerve tissue, the brain, the adrenal glands, liver, kidneys and in mother's milk. In fact, your liver makes the quantity of cholesterol your body

needs to synthesise and transport certain hormones throughout your body. In excess, however, cholesterol becomes far less benign. It is a major part of the common gallstone, is found in many cysts, in some cancerous tissue and is also the fatty deposit found in atheroma.

Simply put, excess cholesterol is responsible for much of the narrowing that occurs in atherosclerosis and most of it gets there because we eat it. Very large quantities of cholesterol are present in the saturated fat products we consume. In fact, all of the cholesterol in your diet comes from foods of animal origin such as meat, fish, fowl, milk, cheese, butter and eggs.

A surplus of cholesterol in the diet causes fatty streaks to appear in the blood – even of people who appear slim and healthy. Given time, this fatty substance adheres to the lining of the arteries and effectively narrows them, especially at points where the lining is already damaged. You know the rest of the story: narrowed arteries can cause hypertension, blood clots, angina, heart attack and stroke. You can see that the quantity of saturated fats and cholesterol in your diet determines, to a large extent, your chances of suffering from cardiovascular disease. The solution seems equally clear:

- reduce your intake of *all* fats
- reduce your intake of saturated fat
- reduce levels of cholesterol in your diet to a maximum of 200 milligrams per day

The most immediate and straightforward means of accomplishing these three goals is to **avoid all animal products**, but if this is too drastic, a good start will be made if you *cut down* your intake of animal products, especially the red meats (beef, lamb, pork), as much as possible. Eat white meats in preference, or fish, but reduce the usual quantities and cook them in a sensible way (see page 00).

SALT
Most of us consume an excess of sodium chloride, better known to us as salt. Whereas healthy adults need only 1.1 to 1.3 grams of sodium per day (maximum), many of us consume four to five times this quantity each day and some people are known to consume *twenty times* this amount! Taken on a regular basis, these quantities can cause an imbalance in the sodium/potassium ratio in your body and health problems may follow. Excess

sodium in the diet is more common than excess potassium and it creates health problems because it promotes fluid retention.

Among these problems are headaches, pre-menstrual tension, swelling of the feet and ankles, possible kidney disorders and high blood pressure. A reduction in your salt intake will help to minimize your risk from these problems. Black people and those persons with a family history of high blood pressure are particularly vulnerable to the health risks from a high-salt diet. However, all of us should take a close look at our own intake of salt to ensure that it is not excessive. In fact, about one-third of your sodium intake probably comes from eating processed foods like salty snacks and tinned foods. Another third of your intake is self-administered as happens when you add salt in cooking or to your individual serving; and a final third is present in high-salt foods such as these listed below:

Soy Sauce	Baking Powder
Baking Soda	Meat
Poultry	Dairy Foods
Seafood	Pickles
Sauces	Stock Cubes & Extracts

By avoiding high-salt foods and by limiting the amounts of salt you add to your food, you may drastically reduce your risk from high blood pressure. There are many salt substitutes available to liven up the taste of your meals, many of which have been used for centuries. My favourites are herbs, spices, celery seeds and lemon juice. And when I really want the flavour of salt, I use Biosalt (TM)[2] which is a compound of tissue salts that are balanced to benefit your body.

If you have a craving for salty foods, try taking a zinc supplement: it may depress your craving which was possibly caused by zinc deficiency in the first place. At the same time, you may wish to increase your intake of potassium by eating potassium-rich foods such as bananas, oranges, whole grains, green leafy vegetables, sunflower seeds and potatoes in their skins.

SUGAR

People often say that sugar is necessary to give you energy and, to an extent, they are right. Sugar is a natural by-product of the

[2] Biosalt (TM) is produced by Gilbert's Health Foods Ltd., Marfleet, Kingston upon Hull, HU9 5NJ, England.

digestive process and it does supply energy by converting the carbohydrate group of foods into starches and glucose (blood sugar). But sugar which is refined, as from sugar beet or sugar cane, is an unnecessary addition to your diet, one that may create long-term health problems.

A diet full of sweets, soft drinks and sweetened teas and coffees undermines your health by laying the foundations for obesity, arthritis, asthma, diabetes, dental decay and cardiovascular disease. It robs your body of an important vitamin (the B-complex), supplies too many 'empty' calories and creates imbalance in the ratio of calcium to phosphorus, so important to the health of your bones and teeth.

COMPLEX CARBOHYDRATES & FIBRE

Carbohydrates are either simple or complex. Simple carbohydrates are found in such foods as sugar and fruits. These carbohydrates provide instant energy to the body in the form of glucose (blood sugar). The simple carbohydrates are often, but not always, high in calories and low in nutrients. They should be eaten in moderate amounts.

Complex carbohydrates, or starches, are found in vegetables, fruits, whole grains, seeds and nuts. These foods usually have a low calorie-to-bulk ratio and should make up the greater portion of your diet. Complex carbohydrates are slowly broken down in the gut to supply a steady trickle of glucose into your bloodstream. A diet that is two-thirds complex carbohydrate is beneficial and may minimize or reverse some of the ill-effects of an earlier, unhealthy diet. Complex carbohydrates also contain cellulose, or fibre.

A high-fibre diet creates a feeling of 'fullness' so that, in terms of calories, you derive more satisfaction from less food. Therefore, a high-fibre diet is important in the prevention of obesity and the maintenance of correct weight. Diets high in fibre also reduce the incidence and the risk of cardiovascular disease as the two types of fibre – soluble and insoluble – act together to alter levels of glucose and cholesterol in your blood.

A high-insoluble fibre diet slows down the digestive process so that more nutrients may be absorbed from your food. Also, the breakdown of food into glucose is more gradual so great surges in your blood sugar level are avoided. Such surges place a great deal of stress on the body and therefore contribute to cardiovascular risk. While digestion is slowed, the limination process is speeded up when you consume a high-fibre diet. Insoluble fibre absorbs water, toxins and food residues as it moves through your digestive system and eases the passage of waste through your bowel.

Soluble fibre is digestible and is commonly described as the 'gel' or 'gum' of carbohydrate foods. It is thought that soluble fibre encourages the body to excrete excess cholesterol. The effect is a lower blood cholesterol level and a simultaneous reduction in your risk from atheroma and the cardiovascular disease associated with it. This list of foods will help you to increase your intake of fibre, both soluble and insoluble, and decrease your risk from cardiovascular disease at the same time:

High-Fibre Foods	No or Low-Fibre Foods
Whole Grains	Meat
Beans & Pulses	Fish
Raw Fruits	Fowl
Vegetables – raw or lightly cooked	Milk & Cheese
Nuts & Sweets	Eggs
Wholewheat Pasta	White Bread
Wholewheat Bread	Polished Rice
	Refined Flour Foods

TEA AND COFFEE

While the occasional cup of tea or coffe may be uplifting and pleasant, regular use of either beverage may increase your risk of suffering cardiovascular disease. This relationship is not confirmed and is not considered a major factor in the reduction or risk. However, three points are worth thinking about:

1) tea and coffee may increase feelings of stress, which is known to raise blood pressure and cholesterol levels in some people.
2) many people have a cigarette at the same time as they drink their tea or coffee. Smoking is known to cause cardiovascular disease. Might a reduction in smoking occur with reduced coffee intake?
3) cream is high in saturated fat and cholesterol; many people add it to their coffee or tea. Reduced tea or coffee intake would reduce saturated fat and cholesterol intake as a result.

If you can't eliminate these drinks from your diet, at least try and reduce your intake to a maximum of two or three cups per day. There are many herbal teas and cereal 'coffees' on the market which you may use instead.

ESSENTIAL NUTRIENTS

Apart from supplying you with energy, your food must also supply the vitamins and minerals your body needs to function at its best. Here is a summary of how various nutrients act on your body and how they may affect your cardiovascular health.

Vitamins

Vitamins are organic substance found in all living things. They are necessary for growth and maintenance of health throughout one's life. Vitamins do not supply energy, they contain no calories, but they are essential for the proper functioning of all your body's systems. Most vitamins are available only through your diet.

There are two basic forms of vitamin water-soluble and fat-soluble. Water-soluble vitamins are easily lost in cooking, cutting, aging and washing of the particular food. They are not stored in your body and so they must be taken frequently if the recommended requirements are to be met. Fat-soluble vitamins are lost in heat, light, air and cooking. They are stored in the fatty tissues of your body and so excess doses may cause toxic reactions.

- Vitamin A is a fat-soluble vitamin essential for the continuous repair and replacement of cell tissues throughout your body. It is present in two forms: carotene and retinol (pre-formed). Carotene is available in fresh vegetables of a dark green leafy nature and those, such as carrots and pumpkin, that have a deep golden colour. The body converts some of the carotene in these vegetables into pre-formed vitamin A (retinol), which is stored in your liver, kidneys, lungs and eyes.
- Vitamin B is really a group of vitamins, often called the vitamin B complex. It consists of more than twelve different water-soluble substances which maintain the health of your nervous system, your blood and your circulatory system. This group is known for reducing the physical consequences of stress – which makes it particularly important for those who already suffer from high cholesterol levels, hypertension and angina. In fact, one particular vitamin from this group, Niacin (B3), is used medically to reduce the level of serum cholesterol

66

in people who have already suffered a heart attack or who have a genetic tendency to high cholesterol levels.

Although niacin by itself is beneficial, it must be taken in a supplement form to obtain the quantities needed for this cholesterol-lowering effect. The B vitamins need each other in order to function as they should upon the body. For this reason, it is best to obtain your daily supply of the B-complex from your diet, because the B's are presented as a group in your food. You can greatly increase your intake of the B group by adding whole grains, dark green leafy vegetables, seaweed, nuts and seeds to your diet. The B vitamins may also be derived from fungi, fermented foods such as miso or tempeh, and yeast products.

- Vitamin C is another water-soluble vitamin which is crucial to the formation of strong cells, especially red blood cells. This vitamin prevents excessive swelling, bleeding and pain which can be caused by the breakdown of red blood cells and also provides resistance to infection.

Also called ascorbic acid, this vitamin is present in most fresh fruits and vegetables, but citrus fruit, green peppers, alfalfa sprouts, broccoli and tomatoes are particulary rich sources. Light, heat, age and air reduce the vitamin C content of food. Fresh fruits and vegetables should be eaten daily as vitamin C is not stored in the body for longer than three or four hours. It is best to obtain your supply of this vitamin from your diet and to 'top up' during stressful times using a dietary supplement.

- Vitamin D is a fat-soluble vitamin derived, in part, from exposure to the sun. A fatty substance in your skin, dehydro-cholesterol, reacts with the sunlight to manufacture vitamin D, which improves your ability to abosrb calcium and phosphorus. Both of these minerals are essential for strong bones and teeth, a stable nervous system and normal blood clotting and heart action.
- Vitamin E is a fat-soluble vitamin which protects red blood cells, improves their capacity to transport oxygen and prevents impaired flow of blood through clotting. It enhances the action of other major nutrients by preventing them from breaking down before your body can use them This break down is called oxidation, therefore vitamin E is an anti-oxidant. It is essential in the process of nourishing and preserving the health of cells, especially blood cells, and enhances your body's ability to withstand pollutants. A

deficiency of vitamin E (as well as vitamins B and C) might create the conditions necessary for a stroke. Vitamin E is available in cold-pressed plant oils, wheat-germ, nuts, seeds and soybeans.

- Vitamin F is the name given to all three 'essential' fatty acids: linoleic, linolenic and arachidonic. These fatty acids must be obtained from your diet because your body cannot make them for itself. Vitamin F assists in the transport and effectiveness of the other fat-soluble vitamins and improves the transport of oxygen through the blood to all your body tissues. Thus the overall health of your tissues and the efficiency of your blood is improved.

Foods which contain the essential fatty acids are the cold-pressed vegetable oils such as safflower oil, soybean oil and corn oil, as well as raw seeds, njts and wheat-germ. These foods are easy to obtain, supply significant amounts of vitamin F, and are healthy substitutes for saturated fat products.

Minerals

Minerals are both organic and inorganic substances which must be taken in the diet. They are needed to build and sustain your body because every tissue in the body contains minerals and every bodily process and action requires minerals. Minerals act with other minerals and with vitamins; deficiencies not corrected by dietary changes can result in illness.

- Calcium is a mineral which helps in the process of normal blood clotting, in nerve function and in the formation of healthy bones and teeth. It is available in a great many foods but needs to be present in company with Phosphorus, Magnesium and Iron, as well as the fat-soluble vitamins (A, D, E), in order for your body to use it well.

Only about 25 per cent of the calcium you take in is abosrbed by your body and, surprisingly, you need more of this mineral as you get older because your body's ability to absorb it decreases with age. Calcium is present in molasses, soya products, seaweed, dried fruits, almonds, celery, dark green leafy vegetables, kale and a great many other delicious foods. For maximum benefit, calcium foods are best eaten separate from starchy food. Also, avoid chocolate, rhubarb and spinach if you know you have a calcium deficiency.

- Iron combines with protein the body and, when further combined with copper, creates haemoglobin. Iron helps many of the vitamins and mineals do their work and builds your resistance to infection and disease. Get your supply of iron from dried fruits, whole grains, dark green leavy vegetables and by cooking in an iron pot!

- Magnesium helps convert glucose to energy, helps in the breakdown of carbohydrate and protein, helps your body make use of other minerals and vitamins and generally plays a crucial role in how your body metabolizes. Magnesium is important in the development of bones, teeth, muscle and nerve and affects the strength of your heart and artery walls.

It is difficult to find a plant food that does not supply magnesium, but whole grains, seaweeds, nuts, dark green leafy vegetables and molasses are particularly good sources. Your body usually absorbs the magnesium it requires from your diet; however, if you are using a diuretic, a hormone drug or consume a lot of alcohol, you would do well to supplement the magnesium in your diet. This mineral is usually present in the mult-mineral tablets currently available on the market.

- Phosphorus is present in every cell in your body and is used in nearly every function your body performs, including repair and metabolisation of food. It is particularly important in the contraction of muscles, even those you don't see, such as the heart. Phosphorus is found in seeds, whole grains, beans, lentils and nuts.
- Potassium is a mineral which works together with sodium to balance the fluid inside and outside the cells walls. Your heart, nerves, kidneys and skin rely on an adequate supply of potassium, but all metabolic processes require that it be present in correct proportions with sodium. Magnesium helps maintain healthy levels of potassium. Potatoes, bananas, oranges, sunflower seeds and green, leafy vegetables provide excellent sources of potassium. Alcohol, sugar and coffee deplete supplies of potassium as does a high intake of sodium.
- Zinc is a wonderful mineral that is still revealing its uses and affiliations within the body. However, in terms of cardio-vascular disease, it is known to be useful in the excretion of cholesterol and in the treatment of atherosclerosis. It also helps to promote healing of internal wounds and damaged arteries. Yeast products, whole grains and seeds are tasty foods with useful quantities of zinc, especially if they have been organically grown.

A VERY SIMPLE SOLUTION

To minimize your risk from cardiovascular disease and, at the same time, maximize your potential for general good health, follow this five-point diet plan:

1) Eat minimal amounts of animal produce
2) Eat minimal amounts of fat
3) Eat minimal amounts of sodium
4) Increase your fibre intake
5) Eat unprocessed, organic food when possible.

Reductions in the amount of sugar, alcohol, tea and coffee you consume will also benefit your health. But health doesn't really mean that you constantly 'give things up'. There are hundreds of foods that fit happily into this five-point plan which are delicious, easy to prepare, attractive, healthy and inexpensive. Let's move on now to the more positive, creative and edible features of a diet that will ensure you keep a healthy heart.

CHAPTER SIX

The Healthy Heart Diet

In this chapter I would like to summarize the features of diet and lifestyle that benefit your cardiovascular health. We have looked into these features, and their negative counterparts, in the previous chapters – now it is time to act on this information to establish a diet and lifestyle that will create long-term health for you and your children.

CHANGES

Diet is usually the habit of a lifetime and yours has probably developed from your environment and your upbringing. Yet it is likely that, in order to improve your health, you will need to break this habit and make changes in what you eat. Any sort of change can be difficult to manage at times, but, in fact, this change can be fun! There is so much to learn about the foods you will be eating, so much to learn about health, nutrition, cookery methods and food presentation. If you welcome this break from old dietary habits, you could discover new, creative talents in yourself.

HOW YOU WILL BENEFIT

Let me remind you of how the cardiovascular diseases are improved or prevented.

- Obesity contributes to cardiovascular disease and is reversed by avoiding animal products as much as possible, as well as alcohol and sugar, and by increasing your fibre intake and your level of exercise.
- Hypertension is reduced or prevented when you quit smoking, cut down on sodium and alcohol consumption and increase your fibre intake and level of exercise.
- Atherosclerosis is reversed or prevented by reducing your fat and animal produce consumption, increasing your fibre intake and level of exercise and quitting smoking.

- Angina is improved or prevented by making all the dietary changes recommended in this book. At the same time, you should increase your level of exercise and attend to your way of dealing with stress.
- Heart attacks are a sign of advanced cardiovascular disease and are best prevented by adjusting both your diet and your lifestyle according to these recommendations. The early you make this adjustment, the better the your long-term health prospects.
- Stroke is a cerebrovascular accident which, nonetheless, has a disease process similar, in its early stages, to cardiovascular disease. High blood pressure and atherosclerosis may contribute to this event. Adjust your diet and lifestyle according to the recommendations listed for these disorders.

ACTION ON LIFESTYLE

Here are the summary guidelines for a healthy heart lifestyle:

- Moderate alcohol consumption – as laid down in chapter 4.
- Weight to be kept within the limits established for optimum health, according to height, gender and frame. (See page 47 for relevant charts.)
- Stop smoking. (See page 50 for useful tips on quitting.)
- Learn to control the level of stress you feel.
- Exercise regularly – at least three times each week for 20 to 30 minutes each session.
- If you are a woman using the contraceptive pill, have regular visits with your doctor to monitor blood pressure.
- The most important change of lifestyle you can make, however, is to make these and the dietary changes *permanent*. Make them into new habits that will bring you good health for the rest of your life.

ACTION ON DIET

Here are the summary guidelines for the healthy heart diet:

- Fat consumption should be reduced so that a maximum of 25% of your total calorie intake is from fats. A simple way to do this is by cutting your current intake in half!
- Cholesterol in your diet should be reduced by avoiding saturated fat and all animal products (including meat, eggs, milk and cheese) as much as possible. Ideally, your cholesterol

should measure less than 5mmols/litre. A reading higher than this means that you should make changes in your diet. Make an appointment today to have your cholesterol tested.

- Salt consumption in this country is between five and twenty times what is adequate and healthy. Avoid salty foods and snacks, and use a salt alternative in cooking and as a condiment to your meals. A sodium intake of 1.1 to 1.3 grams per day is adequate for health.
- Sugar consumption should be drastically reduced. Naturally sweet foods, such as fruit, should be eaten instead of refined sugars.
- Fibre in your diet is known to help reduce weight, improve your overall health and decrease the level of cholesterol in your blood. Increase your consumption of high-fibre, complex carbohydrate foods to comprise 60–70% of your diet.
- Tea and coffee should be consumed in moderation to minimize stress. Drink them without sugar and use soya milk instead of cream.
- Vitamins and minerals are nutrients that maintain and improve your health. Ensure that your food is rich in nutrients by eating as much fresh, unprocessed food as possible.

ACTION FOR LIFE

This four-point plan combines lifestyle and diet. If you value your health and wish to prevent cardiovascular disease and disaster for yourself and your family, adopt this first step in preventative medicine.

1) Limit your eating of animal produce as much as possible
2) Start eating high-fibre foods
3) Stop smoking
4) Start exercising regularly

WELCOMING THE HEALTHY HEART DIET

These simple steps will enable you to prepare yourself, your family and your kitchen for healthy heart diet. Take up to one week to move gradually into these changes.

- First, make public your decision to improve your health. Tell your family, friends and even your colleagues at work. They will encourage you over the next few weeks and they'll also be interested in how you feel and what you eat.

- Make an appointment with your doctor *this week* to have your blood pressure and your serum cholesterol measured. Make a record of these readings and keep it in a safe place for future reference. Both tests are quick to perform and give immediate results.
- If you have a set of scales at home, weight yourself and make a record of your weight, the day of the week and the time of day. Also note whether you weighed yourself with or without shoes and clothing. Place this record in a safe place and weigh yourself each week on the same day and at approximately the same time. Keep a record of your weight changes, if you like.
- Gradually reduce the stock of food in your cupboards and refrigerator to eliminate those foods which will not benefit your cardiovascular health.

- Restock your cupboards with only those foods which will actively enhance your cardiovascular health. Foods to include:

Fruits: Fresh fruits or fruit juices and unsweetened tinned tinned and frozen fruits may be eaten by themselves or as part of a dessert, breakfast or beverage. Dried fruits, especially sundried, may be carried as a between-meals snack, used in sugarless cakes, in muesil or as a sweetener in favoury dishes.

Vegetables: Fresh, organic and in-season vegetables are the most nutritious and therefore most beneficial to health. They are a major component of salads, casseroles, soups and most savoury dishes. The preparation methods which help to retain the nutritional value of vegetables are those which use the vegetable raw, steamed, new-sauted, grilled and baked.

Grains, Legumes, Nuts & Seeds: Unrefined these are the backbone of the healthy heart diet. They are available all the year round and supply very basic nutritional needs in quantity. Foods from this group should always be purchased whole and unprocessed. So, for instance, brown rice instead of polished rice, raw nuts and seeds instead of roasted or salted, and all members of the group organically grown if possible.

NOTE: These first three food groups provide the high-fibre, low-fat features of your diet.

Eggs & Dairy Products: If you can, avoid all the dairy foods, particularly cream and butter. Use skimmed milk or best, soya milk (now available in most of the supermarkets). Use low-fat, natural yogurt or, better, soft tofu (soya cheese); instead of lard or cream cheese, use low-fat cottage cheeses, quark or, again best, firm tofu. However, low-fat the dairy products may be, they *still* contain fat and cholesterol, so the alternatives will always be better. Several brands of egg replacer are widely available when you want the binding or whipping characteristics of egg.

Meat: Cut down on your meat, fish and fowl intake – or avoid it if you can – and, instead, explore the wider range of vegetable proteins available on the market. These include numerous brands of vegetable burgers, texturized vegetable protein (TVP) in the form of mince and chunks, soya cheese, tofu, and the delcious soybean 'meat' from Indonesia called tempeh.

Sugar: Dried fruits, fruit juices and fresh fruit all provide a naturally sweet taste. If you want to use something stronger in flavour try molasses. It is tasty, versatile and high in nutrients.

Salt: Use lemon juice, celery seed, herbs and spices instead of salt. For a healthy, but salty tasting, alternative try Biosalt (TM) which is a chemically balanced blend of salts conducive to your good health.

You should find that your local supermarket stocks most of these food items, as they have become much more popular in recent years. However, if you cannot find one or two foods, or if you simply wish to explore the range of foods available, visit your nearest whole food shop. Most small towns now have a whole food shop and the proprietors are usually quite knowledgeable and friendly.

PREPARING THE HEALTHY HEART DIET

Here are guidelines for healthy preparation of healthy food. These will ensure that the food you buy remains as nutritious as possible until the moment you eat it.

Utensils

- There are two kitchen utensils that are very useful for making the change to healthy cooking. They are a *universal steamer* and a *pressure cooker*. Steaming is an alternative to boiling vegetables, it is as quick as boiling but leaves more of the flavour and nutrition in your food. A Universal Steamer is sold for only two or three pounds.

A pressure cooker is a quick and efficient way of cooking beans and pulses while keeping their nutritional value. Food is cooked with very little water in a sealed pan so that the steam created is kept under pressure. Vegetables may also be cooked in this way, although the saving in time is not nearly so great as with cooking beans. A stainless steel pressure cooker is preferable to an aluminium version and will cost several pounds. Your next birthday present?

I will take this opportunity to recommend that you gradually eliminate your stock of aluminium pans – unless they are enamel coated. Aluminium is known to be toxic to the human body and, unfortunately, pans made from this metal have recently been shown to pass some toxicity into the foods they contain. Instead, use stainless steel, enamel coated, glass or iron pans. Non-stick pans are also recommended, espcially as they help reduce the quantity of oil needed in cooking.

Cooking Methods

The way you cook your food is often as important to its ultimate nutritional value as the type of food you buy in the first place. Many cookery methods cause great loss of nutrients and some methods even turn a healthy food into an unhealthy one. Here are methods which preserve the quality of your food.

- STEAMING: Use a universal steamer, as described above, to cook your vegetables quickly but without losing nutrients or texture. For istance, broccoli, cauliflower, carrots and even potatoes retain their colour, shape, 'biting' texture and flavour – all the qualities that used to end up in the water they are boiled in.
- SAUTÉ: This method is often crucial in order to bring out the aroma and flavour of onions, garlic and some vegetables and it will be used in this diet. However, two distinct forms of sauté are recommended.

In the *Half Sauté* method a *maximum* of only 15ml (1 tbsp) of oil is used. The oil must be one of the oils high in linoleic acid, such as sunflower, safflower, corn, soya or olive. It should be measured into the pan and heated over a medium to high heat (not smoking or spitting) before the food stuff is added. Stir the food constantly, adding other foods as per the recipe. Keep the heat high until the juice from the foods are released into the oil. Then reduce the heat and add any liquid etc. that is required. This method ensures the quality of flavour and aroma desired from a sauté, as well as the reduction in fat needed for health.

The *New Sauté* method does not use oil but still achieves the flavour, aroma, texture and nutritional quality desired from the sauté stage of cooking. Instead, of oil, a very small amount (usually 15–30 ml (1–2 Tbsp)) of liquid is heated in the pan until it bubbles furiously. The liquid may be water, stock, tomato juice, vinegar, gravy broth, dilute yeast extract or, indeed, any liquid you wish to use. Once the liquid is heated, the food is added and stirred constantly over a medium to high heat. As the food is more likely to stick in this method, the saute time is not so long and the heat is slightly higher than in the oil sauté.

- FRYING: Fried food is not recommended.
- BOILING: Rice and beans may be boiled and some sauces and soups may be brought to a boil before reducing them to a simmer. However, boiling is not usually used to cook vegetables as if greatly reduces their nutritional value and may cause them to lose texture, colour and flavour.
- GRILLING: This method of cooking greatly reduces or eliminates the use of oil and fat in cooking.
- OVEN BAKING: A few of the recipes included make use of the oven. If little fat is used, baked foods can retain much of their nutritional value – a baked jacket potatato is full of goodness!
- RAW: Most of the foods you will eat may be eaten raw. With a few exceptions (such as cooked carrot), raw food is nutritionally richer than its cooked counterpart and often has much more flavour. Buy organically grown foods when possible, especially fruits and vegetables. Raw foods are opportunities for you to create visual interest in your meal according to how you slice, shred, tear and chop them. And because they can be very colourful, you may wish to bring out the artist in you and serve them in dishes of unusual shapes and colours.
- COOKING BROWN RICE: 450g (1 lb) is equal to 2 full cups of raw brown rice. Rice is cooked in twice its volume of water, therefore one pound of rice needs to cook in 4 cups (2 pints) of water. Rice trebles in bulk when cooked to make approximately 6 cupsful of cooked rice. This is enough to serve four people when a sauce or savoury accompanies the rice.

Method: Measure the rice into a mixing bowl and cover with cold water. Now wash the rice by swirling your hand through it and exerting a scrubbing motion. Drain the water and repeat this process three times until the water is fairly clear. Drain the rice and tip into an iron pot.

When cooking rice, the ratio of water to rice is generally 2/1.

Cover the clean rice in the pan with twice its volume in water. Cover the pan and place over a high flame. Bring the water to the boil, then reduce the flame as much as possible and leave to simmer for approximately 50 minutes or until the water is completely absorbed. Keep the pan covered while it cooks, only lifting the lid at the end of the cooking time to check that the rice is finished.

Don't stir the rice at this point, or it may become gummy. If it is still too firm at the end of 50 minutes, boil the kettle and add a little boiling water to the rice. Cover again and cook for another 10 minutes.

Brown rice takes longer to cook than white rice because it is a whole grain. However, it is more nutritious than white, refined rice and has ten times the flavour.

- COOKING BEANS: Most beans doube in bulk once they are cooked. To gauge how much you need for a meal, the rule of thumb is that 55–155g (2–4oz) of dried beans are enough for one serving, depending on what will accompany them. All beans must be well washed and well cooked to avoid flatulence.

Method: Measure the beans into a mixing bowl and pick them over to remove any stones or unwanted pieces of bean.

Cover the beans with cold water and wash them very well by swirling your hand through them and exerting a scrubbing motion. Pour the water away and repeat this process three times, or until the water is clear. Drain the beans.

Cover the beans with water and leave them to soak overnight or all day while you are at work. Soaking the beans helps to prevent the flatulence that some people suffering from eating beans.

Drain the beans and throw the water away. Tip the beans into an iron pot and cover them with water. Bring them to the boil and simmer with the pan partially covered for 1–3 hours, depending on the type of bean you are cooking. The beans must remain covered in water and they must cook until they are easily squashed between your tongue and the top of your mouth. If they are under-cooked you will get a stomach ache.

Alternatively, some beans may be pressure cooked. Cover the beans with water, cover the cooker and bring up to pressure. Cook at pressure for 20–40 minutes, depending on the type of bean you are cooking. (Please refer to the leaflet accompanying your pressure cooker.)

In both methods, adding a strip of Kombu (seaweed) to the water will help to soften the beans.

Red Lentils and Split Peas do not require soaking or pressure cooking. They do require washing. The red lentils are especially quick to cook and are therefore very useful for a quick, nutritious 'complete protein' meal.

Chickpeas: Take 30 minutes in the pressure cooker; 3 hours in the pot.

Kidney Beans: Take 30 minutes in the pressure cooker; 1½ hours in the pot.

Butter Beans: Take 30 minutes in the pressure cooker; 1½ hours in the pot.

Soybeans: TAke 40 minutes in the pressure cooker; at least 3 hours in the pot.

Blacked-eyed Beans: Take 20 minutes in the pressure cooker; 1 hour in the pot.

Lentils & Split Peas: Take 20 minutes in the pressure cooker; 1 hour in the pot.

NUTRITIONAL ANALYSIS

Each of the recipes in the next section has been analysed to give their nutritional value in seven important aras:

calories – important in weight control
fibre – important in weight contrlol and cholesterol reduction
total fat – important in weight control and atherosclerosis
saturated fat – a factor in atherosclerosis and high cholesterol
unsaturated fat – may help reduce cholesterol level and weight
cholesterol – contribute to atherosclerosis and heart attack
sodium – a factor in hypertension

In order to use these analyses to your advantage, compare your daily intake in these seven areas with the recommended daily intake for your gender. These figures are approximate recommended daily intakes for a modrately active adult over the age of 22 years. These figures do not apply and are not appropriate for children, adolscents or for pregnant or nursing mothers.

	ADULT MALE	ADULT FEAMLE
Calories	2600	2000
Fibre	25–45 grams	25–45 grams
Total Fat	maximum 72 grams	maximum 56 grams
Saturated Fat	maximum 29 grams	maximum 22 grams
Unsaturated Fat	maximum 43 grams	maximum 34 grams
Cholesterol	maximum 200 mg	maximum 200 mg
Sodium	1.1–1.3 grams	1.1–1.3 grams

Now you are ready to begin the healthy heart diet. Remember to weight yourself each week and to keep a record of any weight reduction. Then, after a minimum of one month, but no later than six months from now, return to your doctor and have your blood pressure and serum cholesterol measured again. Compared these readings to your first test to see the positive effects of your change in diet and lifestyle.

CHAPTER SEVEN

Healthy Heat Recipes

The majority of the recipes in this chapter will make high-fibre, low-fat, low-sodium meals, which are free of all animal products. Each recipe is accompanied by a nutritional analysis which gives values for calories, total fat, saturated fat, unsaturated fat, cholesterol, fibre and sodium. These figures are taken from the Expanded Foods Database, Nutri-Calc Plus (TM)[1]. They are based on nutritional analyses that are currently available, therefore many of the figures are approximate. Please note that the figures given for fibre are for crude, or insoluble, fibre only.

However, I have included a few recipes using animal products – the less fatty white meats, white fish, milk, cheese and yoghurt. These are for those of you reluctant to cut out animal products completely. Although they are 'healthy' in that they cut out undesirables like butter and cream, and have reduced quantities of meats, a quick comparison with the nutritional analyses of the other recipes will show that they are much less basically healthy than those *not* using animal products.

Most of the recipes serve four people, but a few serve more or less people so be sure to check the number of servings recommended. The analyses are listed per portion, unless otherwise stated, i.e. Value for Whole Cake or Total Value. In these cases, divide the figures by the number of servings you decide the recipe will make.

[1]based on nutritional figures from the U.S. Department of Agriculture Handbook 8 and food manufacturers' analyses.

SOUPS

Norwegian Potato Soup

Serves 4
Value Per Portion: Calories 223
Total Fat: 516 gm   Saturated Fat: 102 gm
Unsaturated Fat: 27 gm   Cholesterol: 0 mg
Fibre: 1.429 gm   Sodium 54.74 mg

1 kilo (2 lb) potatoes
2 medium sized onions
30ml (2 tbsp) cider vinegar
5–10ml (1–2 tsp) freshly ground black pepper
5ml (1 tsp) caraway seed
1–2 litres (3–4 pints) water
5 stalks celery
3 bays leaves

Scrub and dice the potatoes then place them in a colander and rinse them under cold water. Leave to drain. Finely chop the onions and sauté them in the vinegar. Use a large, deep saucepan and stir constantly over a medium flame. When the onions are soft, add the potatoes, pepper and caraway. Stir well then add the water and keep stirring for 1–2 minutes. Bring the soup to a low boil, reduce the heat and simmer, covered, for 20 minutes. Chop the celery and add to the soup. Add the bay leaves. Simmer for a further 10–15 minutes and serve.

Courgette and Tofu Soup

Serves 4
Value Per Portion: Calories: 53.19
Total Fat: 1.438 gm   Saturated Fat: .034 gm
Unsaturated Fat: .099 gm   Cholesterol: 0 mg
Fibre: .698 gm   Sodium: 12.16 mg

4 small courgettes
115g (4 oz) firm tofu
1 medium onion
1 litre (approx. 2 pints) water
140g (5 oz) tomato puree
2.5ml (½ tsp) freshly ground black pepper
5ml (1 tsp) dried basil

Wash the courgettes: trim them then slice them into thin rounds. Drain the tofu and cut into small cubes. Peel and thinly slice the onion. Mix the water and tomato puree together in a jug then stir in the black pepper and basil. Place a large saucepan over a medium flame and heat it for two or three minutes. Then pour approximately 60ml (2 fl.oz) of the tomato sauce into the pan so that it bubbles immediately. Drop the onion into the sauce and stir constantly as you would a sauté. Add more sauce if necessary. When the onions have softened, add the courgettes and continue to stir over a medium to high heat for three minutes. Add the remaining sauce, stir well and cover the pan. Reduce the heat and leave it to simmer gently for 15 minutes. Add the tofu, stir the soup and leave it over the heat for a further 5 minutes. Serve hot.

Athenian Carrot Soup

Serves 4
Value Per Portion:
Total Fat: 2.93 gm
Unsaturated Fat: 1.861 gm
Fibre: 3.686 gm

Calories: 256
Saturated Fat: .345 gm
Cholesterol: 0 mg
Sodium: 321.2 mg

170g (6 oz) dried chickpeas
450g (1 lb) carrots
3 cloves garlic
2 large onions
1 × 425g (15oz) tin chopped tomatoes
5ml (1 tsp) freshly ground black pepper
1–1.5 litres (2–3 pints) water
1 strip of kombu (optional)
15ml (1 tbsp) cider vinegar

Soak, rinse and pressure cook the chickpeas. Scrub the carrots and slice in thin rounds. Finely chop the garlic and onions and sauté them in a large saucepan using a little juice from the tomatoes. Add the ground pepper and carrots to the sauté and stir well. Gradually add the tomatoes and water and bring the mixture to a simmer. Add the kombu and the chickpeas and stir. Simmer for 30 minutes. Just before serving, stir in the vinegar.

Lemon & Lentil Soup

Serves 4
Value Per Portion:
Total Fat: .399 gm
Unsaturated Fat: .234 gm
Fibre: 2.133 gm

Calories: 70.26
Saturated Fat: .044 gm
Cholesterol: 0 mg
Sodium: 7.403 mg

225g (8 oz) dried red lentils
1–1.5 litres (2–3 pints) water
1 small green pepper
1 medium sized fresh chili
juice of 1 lemon

Wash the lentils very well, drain them and add them to the fresh
water in a large saucepan. Bring to the boil, reduce the heat
then cover the pan and simmer for 10 minutes. Wash and chop
the pepper and the chili and add to the lentils. Stir well and
cook for a further 20–30 minutes or until the lentils have
completely lost their shape and are quite mushy. Stir in the
lemon juice just before serving.

Parsley & Celery Soup

Serves 4
Value per Portion:
Total Fat: 3.811 gm
Unsaturated Fat: 3.15 gm
Fibre: 1.279 gm

Calories: 75.63
Saturated Fat: .363 gm
Cholesterol: 0 mg
Sodium: 112.1 mg

15ml (1 tbsp) oil
2 medium onions
5ml (1 tsp) caraway seed
1.5 litres (3 pints) water
1 head celery
1 bunch fresh parsley
juice of 1 orange

Heat the oil in a deep saucepan over a medium flame. Tinly
slice the onions and sauté them until they begin to soften. Then
sprinkle the caraway seed over them and continue to sauté,
stirring constantly. Add the water, stir very well and increase
the flame to bring the broth to a gentle boil. Meanwhile, wash,
trim and chop the celery and parsley. When the broth has boiled,
add the celery and parsley. Stir very well, cover the pan and

reduce the heat. Leave covered and simmer for 10 minutes. Add the orange juice just before serving.

Cream of Broccoli Soup

Serves 4
Value Per Portion:
Total Fat: 12.22 gm
Unsaturated Fat: 3.396 gm
Fibre: 2.649 gm

Calories: 223.7
Saturated Fat: .435 gm
Cholesterol: 0 mg
Sodium: 72.29 mg

15ml (1 tbsp) oil
1 small onion
3 cloves garlic (optional)
10ml (2 tsp) whole wheat flour
570ml (1 pint) soya milk
1 litre (2 pints) water
900g (2 lb) broccoli
5ml (1 tsp) freshly ground black pepper

Heat the oil in a deep enamel saucepan. Finely chop the onion and garlic and sauté over a medium heat for 3 minutes. Sprinkle the flour over the sauté and stir well to make a roux. Mix the soya milk with the water and gradually add to the roux, stirring well after each addition. When all the liquid has been added, reduce the heat and cover the pan. Wash and coarsely chop the broccoli and add to the soup. Add the black pepper and allow the soup to simmer gently for 15–20 minutes, stirring occasionally. You may leave the broccoli in chunks, mash them slightly as you stir, or run the soup through a mouli for an even texture. Serve hot.

White Fish and Leek Soup

Serves 4
Value Per Portion:
Total Fat: 4.179gm
Unsaturated Fat: 3.12gm
Fibre: .723gm

Calories: 142.8
Saturated Fat: .657gm
Cholesterol: 30.63mg
Sodium: 91.88mg

Ingredients:
1 small onion, peeled and thinly sliced
1 garlic clove, peeled and crushed
15 ml (1 tbsp) olive oil

2 medium leeks, washed and cut into thin strips
30ml (2 tbsp) chopped fresh parsley
225g (8 oz) white fish fillet, cubed
285ml (10 fl. oz) vegetable stock
285ml (10 fl. oz) skimmed milk
freshly ground black pepper
15ml (1 tbsp) snipped chives

Sauté the onion and garlic in the olive oil for a few minutes until just softened, then add the leeks and parsley. Continue cooking gently for a few more minutes. Add the cubed fish, stock, milk and seasoning to taste. Bring to the boil and simmer gently for about 10 minutes. Serve hot, garnished with the snipped chives.

SALADS

Grand Fruit Salad

Serves 4
Value Per Portion: Calories: 187.3
Total Fat: 1.068 gm   Saturated Fat: .281 gm
Unsaturated Fat: .35 gm   Cholesterol: 0 mg
Fibre: 1.455 gm   Sodium: 2.632 mg

1 large grapefruit
2 large oranges
1 red eating apple
1 green eating apple
2 ripe bananas
225g (8 oz) seedless grapes
a sprig of fresh mint

Peel the grapefruit and oranges and divide them into segments. Cut the segments roughly in half and place in a large serving bowl. Wash and finely chop the apples and add to the citrus fruits. Peel the bananas, slice them into thin rounds and stir them into the fruit salad. Wash the grapes, pull them from their stalks and add to the salad. Stir the whole very well. Chop the mint coarsely and sprinkle over the fruit salad. Serve immediately or chill for one hour before serving.

October Salad

Serves 4
Value Per Portion: Calories: 186.3
Total Fat: 7.093 gm   Saturated Fat: 1.322 gm
Unsaturated Fat: 5.42 gm   Cholesterol: 0 mg
Fibre: 1.423 gm   Sodium: 64.38 mg

1 large beetroot
¼ head red or white cabbage
15g (½ oz) fresh parsley
4 stalks celery
170g (6 oz) sweetcorn kernals
115g (4 oz) dried currants or sultanas
55g (2 oz) pumpkin or sunflower seeds

Wash, trim and shred the beetroot and cabbage and place them in a large salad bowl. Wash and finely chop the parsley and add to the salad. Thinly slice the celery. Add the celery, sweetcorn, dried fruit and seeds to the salad and stir well. Serve immediately with a vinaigrette or tofu dressing.

Not-the-Waldorf Salad

Serves 4
Value Per Portion: Calories: 286.3
Total Fat: 20.49 gm   Saturated Fat: 1.644 gm
Unsaturated Fat: 15.324 gm   Cholesterol: 0 mg
Fibre: 2.343 gm   Sodium: 27.25 mg

1 small turnip
2 large carrots
1 medium onion
2 eating apples
115g (4 oz) broken walnuts
285g (10 oz) soft tofu
5ml (1 tsp) caraway seeds
juice of half lemon

Wash, trim and shred the turnip and carrots and place them in a salad bowl. Peel the onion; finely chop the onion and apples and add to the salad bowl. Add the remaining ingredients to the salad and stir well. Serve slightly chilled with a garnish of parsley or lemon peel.

Hot Potato Salad

Serves 4
Value Per Portion:

Total Fat: 3.748 gm	Calories: 245.7
Unsaturated Fat: 2.874 gm	Saturated Fat: .515 gm
Fibre: 1.074 gm	Cholesterol: 0 mg
	Sodium: 35.49 mg

900g (2 lb) new potatoes
¼ head white cabbage
3 cloves garlic
55g (2 oz) fresh parsley
140ml (5 fl oz) cider vinegar
5ml (1 tsp) dry mustard
15ml (1 tbsp) olive oil

Scrub the potatoes and steam them until tender. Finely chop the cabbage and garlic and place in a large serving bowl. Wash and chop the parsley. Mix the remaining ingredients together in a small saucepan and bring to a very gentle simmer. When the potatoes are tender, stir them gently into the cabbage and garlic. Now pour the hot vinaigrette over the salad and stir again. Serve immediately.

Pepper & Pasta Salad

Serves 4
Value Per Portion:

Total Fat: 10.03 gm	Calories: 368.9
Unsaturated Fat: .754 gm	Saturated Fat: .157 gm
Fibre: .503 gm	Cholesterol: 0 mg
	Sodium: 811.8 mg

225g (8 oz) whole wheat pasta shells
1 × 340g (12 oz) tin sweetcorn
1 large green pepper
1 large red pepper
30ml (2 tbsp) chopped chives *or* 2 spring onions

Cook the pasta in a pot of boiling water until just tender, about 12 minutes. Drain well and allow to cool. Pour the sweetcorn into a large salad bowl. Wash and thinly slice the peppers and chives (or onions) and place them in the salad bowl. When it is cool, add the pasta and stir all the ingredients together. Serve with a vinaigrette.

Tomato & Butter Bean Salad

Serves 4
Value Per Portion: Calories: 110.9
Total Fat: .596 gm   Saturated Fat: .127 gm
Unsaturated Fat: .296 gm   Cholesterol: 0 mg
Fibre: 2.29 gm   Sodium: 16.63 mg

115g (4 oz) dried butter beans
4 medium tomatoes
2 small onions
30g (1 oz) fresh parsley
1 sprig fresh mint

Soak, rinse, drain and pressure cook the beans. Allow them to
cool. Coarsely chop the tomatoes and place them in a large
salad bowl. Finely chop the onions, parsley and mint and add
to the tomatoes. Add the cooled beans and stir well. Chill the
salad or serve immediately with a vinaigrette dressing.

Pimento & Onion Salad

Serves 4
Value Per Portion: Calories: 40.75
Total Fat: .275 gm   Saturated Fat: .017 gm
Unsaturated Fat: .06 gm   Cholesterol: 0 mg
Fibre: .408 gm   Sodium: 246.3 mg

115g (4 oz) dried black-eyed beans
1 bunch fresh coriander leaves
1 large sweet onion
juice of 1 lemon
2.5 ml (½ tsp) freshly ground black pepper
50g (2 oz) pimento

Soak the beans and the coriander separately in very cold water
overnight. Rinse, drain and pressure cook the beans. Allow them
to cool. Slice the onion very thinly, break each slice into rings
and place in a large salad bowl. Pour the lemon juice over the
onions and sprinkle with black pepper. Wash and finely chop
the coriander.

Add the pimento, coriander and beans to the onions and stir
together. Serve immediately or chill for later use.

Orange & Almond Salad

Serves 4
Value Per Portion: Calories: 144.1
Total Fat: 4.695 gm   Saturated Fat: .491 gm
Unsaturated Fat: 3.75 gm   Cholesterol: 0 mg
Fibre: 1.22 gm   Sodium: 25.32 mg

450g (1 lb) cooked kidney beans
225g (½ lb) carrots
½ small head white cabbage
2 medium oranges
25g (1 oz) slivered almonds

Ensure the beans are fully cooked (if they are tinned, the label should say if cooking is necessary) and empty them into a large bowl. Shred the carrots and cabbage into the bowl. Peel and thinly slice the oranges and add them, with any juice, to the salad. Sprinkle the almonds over the salad and stir gently. Serve immediately.

Gourmet Garden Salad

Serves 4
Value Per Portion: Calories: 105
Total Fat: .388 gm   Saturated Fat: .064 gm
Unsaturated Fat: .156 gm   Cholesterol: 0 mg
Fibre: 2.719 gm   Sodium: 14.63 mg

680g (1½ pounds) green beans
1 large sweet onion
2 large carrots
2 eating apples

Wash, trim and steam the green beans (15–20 minutes) and allow them to cool. Thinly slice the onion, break each slice into rings and place in a large salad bowl. Grate the carrots and apples into the salad bowl. Stir well and serve immediately.

Chicken Salad

Serves 4
Value Per Portion: Calories: 238.85
Total Fat: 5.03gm   Saturated Fat: 1.357gm
Unsaturated Fat: 2.784gm   Cholesterol 84.6mg
Fibre: 1.32gm   Sodium: 101.5mg

Ingredients:
115g (4 oz) eating apple, cored
15ml (1 tbsp) lemon juice
450g (1 lb) cooked chicken, skinned and cut into strips
115g (4 oz) cucumber, cut into strips
115g (4 oz) fennel, cut into strips
115g (4 oz) red pepper, cored, seeded and cut into strips
1 portion Versatile Fennel Sauce (see page 00)
15ml (1 tbsp) finely chopped parsley

Cut the apple into stripes and toss immediately in the lemon juice. Combine the apple, chicken, cucumber, fennel and red pepper in a mixing bowl. Spoon the sauce over the salad, and sprinkle with the parsley.

MAIN DISHES

Spinach & Mushroom Sauce Over Rice

Serves 4
Value Per Portion:
Total Fat: 2.271 gm
Unsaturated Fat: .321 gm
Fibre: 1.641 gm

Calories: 341.5
Saturated Fat: .11 gm
Cholesterol: 0 mg
Sodium: 779.4

225g (8 oz) whole grain rice
570–710ml (1–1¼ pint) water

Sauce:
1 large onion
225g (8 oz) button mushrooms
30ml (2 tbsp) cider vinegar
270ml (10 fl oz) water
1ml (2 tsp) dried parsley
5ml (1 tsp) dried basil
freshly ground black pepper to taste
450g (1 lb) fresh spinach

Wash the rice three times, drain, place in a large saucepan and cover with the fresh water. Place over a high heat until the water boils. Reduce the heat, cover the pan and simmer the rice, undisturbed, until the water is completely absorbed.

Chop the onion and mushrooms and 'saute' in the vinegar in a deep frying pan. When they are tender, add the water, parsley, basil and pepper and stir over a medium heat. When the liquid simmers, cover the pan and reduce the heat. Wash and drain the spinach then trim it and chop it coarsely. Pack the spinach into the frying pan with the mushrooms and onions, cover and leave for 15 minutes over a medium heat. At the end of this time, stir the spinach into the sauce and leave over a very low heat until the rice is cooked. Serve the sauce over the rice on heated plates.

Marinated Tofu with Ginger

Serves 4
Value Per Portion:

Total Fat: 3.054 gm	Calories: 78.59
Unsaturated Fat: .207 gm	Saturated Fat: .134 gm
Fibre: .643 gm	Cholesterol: 0 mg
	Sodium: 8.742 mg

285g (10 oz) firm tofu
140ml (5 fl oz) cider vinegar
3g (1 oz) fresh ginger
a pinch of freshly ground black pepper
115g (4 oz) button mushrooms

Cut the tofu into small chunks, place in a bowl and pour the vinegar over. Slice the ginger very thinly and add to the tofu; sprinkle the pepper over it and stir gently. Clean and quarter the mushrooms and add to the tofu, stir again, cover and leave to marinate for 2–4 hours. Serve cold or heat the whole mixture in a saucepan over a medium heat. Serve with rice, pasta or a salad.

Baked Potatoes with Tofu Whip Filling

Serves 4
Value Per Portion:

Total Fat: 2.845 gm	Calories: 281.8
Unsaturated Fat: .155 gm	Saturated Fat: .07 gm
Fibre: 1.568 gm	Cholesterol: 0 mg
	Sodium: 25.75 mg

4 large potatoes
285g (10 oz) soft tofu
1 small onion
1 medium tomato
5ml (1 tsp) dried parsley
10ml (2 tsp) brewer's yeast

Scrub the potatoes, pierce them and bake in a hot oven for 45 minutes, or until well cooked. Mash the tofu in a mixing bowl. Finely chop the onion and tomato and add to the tofu. Add the parsley and yeast and stir the mixture very well. Cut the potatoes in half and spoon one quarter of the tofu whip over each potato. Sprinkle with a little pepper if desired. Serve hot alone or with a salad.

Creamy Pasta and Vegetable Dish

Serves 4

Value Per Portion:

Total Fat: 17.83 gm	Calories: 464.6
Unsaturated Fat: 3.248 gm	Saturated Fat: .372 gm
Fibre: .852 gm	Cholesterol: 0 mg
	Sodium: 1029 mg

225g (8 oz) wholewheat pasta
15ml (1 tbsp) oil
1 medium onion
a pinch of flour
265ml (½ pint) soya milk
2 stalks celery
1 large carrot
285g (10 oz) sweetcorn
15g (½ oz) fresh mint

Cook the pasta in a pot of boiling water until just tender, about 12 minutes. In a separate pan, heat the oil and sauté the finely chopped onion until it is tender. Sprinkle a little flour over the sauté and stir well to make a roux. Then gradually add the soya milk, stirring constantly, to make a sauce. Wash and thinly slice the celery; grate the carrot. Add the celery, carrot and sweetcorn to the sauce and stir well. Chop the mint into the sauce and remove from the heat. Drain the pasta and tip it into a large serving bowl. Pour the sauce over, stir well and serve immediately.

Away All Day Stew

Serves 4
Value Per Portion:
Total Fat: 2.25 gm
Unsaturated Fat: 1.404 gm
Fibre: 8.653 gm

Calories: 614
Saturated Fat: .37 gm
Cholesterol: 0 mg
Sodium: 181.1 mg

455g (1 lb) swedes
455g (1 lb) carrots
455g (1 lb) parsnips
455g (1 lb) turnips
900g (2 lb) potatoes
455g (1 lb) small onions
10ml (2 tsp) whole cloves
12 peppercorns
455g (1 lb) chestnut puree
2 litres (approx. 4 pints) water

Wash and trim or peel the root vegetables and chop them into 2.5cm (1 inch) pieces. Peel the onions and push a whole clove into both ends of each onion. Place all the vegetables and the peppercorns into a large stewpot. Mix the chestnut puree with the water in a jug and, when well mixed, pour over the vegetables. Stir the ingredients well. Cover the pot tightly and place it in the oven at a very low heat – 140°C/275°F (Gas Mark 1) is a perfect setting. If you have an Aga, use the slow oven. Let the stew cook undisturbed for 6–8 hours while you are out at work. Serve hot with fresh bread.

Squash with Herb and Broccoli Filling

Serves 4
Value Per Portion:
Total Fat: 1.084 gm
Unsaturated Fat: .547 gm
Fibre: 2.519 gm

Calories: 80.7
Saturated Fat: .203 gm
Cholesterol: 0 mg
Sodium: 29.91 mg

900g (2 lb) squash
340g (¾ lb) broccoli
30g (1 oz) fresh parsley
3 cloves garlic
1 medium onion

Slice the squash in half lengthwise and remove the seeds. Place each half on a large piece of aluminium foil. Chop the remaining ingredients very finely and blend them together in a mixing bowl. You may add a dash of black pepper if you like. Divide this filling between the two halves of squash and press well down – even so the filling will rise above the edges of the squash. Bring the edges of the aluminium foil up over the filling and fold them together in a seal. Place the filled squash halves together on a roasting tray and bake at 180°C/350°F (Gas Mark 4) for 30–40 minutes. Serve hot with a favourite sauce.

Picnic Marinade

Serves 4
Value Per Portion: Calories: 216.4
Total Fat: 1.524 gm   Saturated Fat: .212 gm
Unsaturated Fat: .894 gm   Cholesterol: 0 mg
Fibre: 4.399 gm   Sodium: 85.88 mg

The Marinade
270ml (½ pint) cider vinegar
juice of 2 lemons
12 whole cloves
12 whole peppercorns
12 cloves of garlic (optional)
5ml (1 tsp) caraway seed
140ml (5 fl oz) apple juice
3 bay leaves
2 small pieces cinnamon
270–450ml (½–¾ pint) water

The Vegetables
225g (½ lb) carrots
340g (12 oz) green beans
1 small red pepper
1 small green pepper
2 small onions
1 medium sized cauliflower
455g (1 lb) broccoli

Gently heat all the marinade ingredients together in a large enamel saucepan while you prepare the vegetables. Note: the cloves of garlic should be peeled but left whole. Wash the vegetables. Thinly slice the carrots, beans, peppers and onions. Cut the cauliflower and broccoli into florets. Simmer all the vegetables in the marinade for 15 minutes. Keep the pan covered but stir occasionally. Remove the pan from the heat, stir the ingredients well, cover the pan and allow the mixture to cool. Serve immediately or chill and eat over the next 3–4 days.

Favourite Tempeh Marinade

Serves 4
Value Per Portion:
Total Fat: 4.435 gm
Unsaturated Fat: .075 gm
Fibre: .39 gm

Calories: 127.6
Saturated Fat: .031 gm
Cholesterol: 0 mg
Sodium: 1.5 mg

225g (8 oz) tempeh
150ml (5 fl oz) cider vinegar
juice of 2 lemons
5ml (1 tsp) mustard seed
12 whole cloves
12 whole peppercorns
3–6 cloves garlic (optional)
2 small onions
1 tart apple

Defrost the tempeh and cut into 1 inch cubes. Place the tempeh in a casserole dish. Mix the vinegar, lemon juice and spices together in a jug. Finely chop the garlic, onions and apple and add to the marinade in the jug. Stir well and pour over the tempeh pieces in the casserole. Cover the casserole and leave the tempeh to marinade for 4–8 hours. Bake, covered, at 180°C/350°F (Gas Mark 4) for 30 minutes. Remove the cover and bake for a further 10 minutes if you want a crispy surface to the tempeh. Serve hot with brown rice and steamed broccoli.

Sweet & Sour Mushrooms over Spaghetti

Serves 4
Value Per Portion:
Total Fat: 1.083 gm
Unsaturated Fat: .15 gm
Fibre: .678 gm

Calories: 254.8
Saturated Fat: .059 gm
Cholesterol: 0 mg
Sodium: 7.556 mg

1 medium sized onion
3 cloves garlic
60ml (2 fl oz) cider vinegar

225g (½ lb) button mushrooms
55g (2 oz) raisins or currants
15ml (1 tbsp) brewer's yeast
5ml (1 tsp) freshly ground black pepper
115g (4 oz) whole wheat spaghetti

Chop onion and garlic and sauté in the vinegar in a large frying pan. Clean and thickly slice the mushrooms and add to the sauté. Stir in the raisins, yeast and pepper, stir well and simmer very gently while you cook the spaghetti. Serve the sauce over the spaghetti.

Ladies' Finger Sauté

Serves 4
Value Per Portion:

Total Fat: 3.833 gm	Calories: 89.52
Unsaturated Fat: 2.967 gm	Saturated Fat: .544 gm
Fibre: 1.565 gm	Cholesterol: 0 mg
	Sodium: 8.53 mg

450g (1 lb) fresh ladies' fingers (okra)
3 cloves garlic
2 small onions
15ml (1 tbsp) olive oil
225g (½ tbsp) olive oil
225 (½ lb) button mushrooms
140–200ml (5–5 fl oz) water

Wash the ladies' fingers and cut off the hard tip of each one. Finely chop the garlic and onion and sauté in the olive oil over a high heat. When they are tender, add the ladies' fingers and stir frequently. Clean the mushrooms and add them to the sauté. Stir well and cook for another 3–4 minutes. Add the water, cover the pan, reduce the heat and cook for 10 minutes longer. Serve immediately with rice, pasta or steamed vegetables.

Scented Rice & Vegetables

Serves 4
Value Per Portion:

Total Fat: 1.805 gm	Calories: 332.2
Unsaturated Fat: .174 gm	Saturated Fat: .053 gm
Fibre: 2.156 gm	Cholesterol: 0 mg
	Sodium: 691.9 mg

Ingredients:
225 (8 oz) whole grain rice
850ml (1.5 pints) water
5ml (1 tsp) turmeric
1 bay leaf
1 × 5cm (2 inch) piece cinnamon
2 small onions
1 small red pepper
1 small green pepper
285g (10 oz) fresh *or* frozen peas

Wash and drain the rice. Bring the water to a low boil and add the turmeric, bay leaf and cinnamon stick. Stir well, then add the rice and bring to the boil again. Cover and simmer for 10 minutes. Finely chop the onions and peppers. Stir the onions, peppers and peas into the cooking rice and cover the pan once more. Cover the pan and cook until the liquid is absorbed. Serve hot or cold.

Brussels Sprouts & Bamboo Shoot Savoury

Serves 4
Value Per Portion:

Calories: 60.36	
Total Fat: .805 gm	Saturated Fat: .166 gm
Unsaturated Fat: .443 gm	Cholesterol: 0 mg
Fibre: 1.913 gm	Sodium: 84.19 mg

5ml (1 tsp) yeast extract
50ml (2 fl oz) water
455g (1 lb) Brussels sprouts
1 small onion
1 × 285 (10 oz) tin bamboo shoots
freshly ground black pepper to taste

Dissolve the yeast extract in the water. Wash and trim the sprouts and halve or quarter them. Chop the onion. rinse the bamboo shoots under cold water and drain. Pour half the yeast into a frying pan and place over a high heat until it begins to bubble. Add the sprouts and onion and stir often for 5 minutes. Add the bamboo shoots and black pepper and stir gently together. Cook for another 5 minutes. Serve over rice, pasta or with other vegetables.

Sweet Potato Bake

Serves 4

Value Per Portion:

Total Fat: .157 gm

Unsaturated Fat: .074 gm

Fibre: 1.066 gm

Calories: 132.9

Saturated Fat: .031 gm

Cholesterol: 0 mg

Sodium: 11.58 mg

450g (1 lb) sweet potatoes
1 large orange
2.5ml (½ tsp) freshly ground black pepper

Scrub the sweet potatoes and quarter them, cutting only ¾ of the way through so that you are able to open them. Lay each potato on a piece of foil *or* arrange them together in a large baking tray. Peel the orange, divide it into segments and cut each segment in half. Place orange pieces in the centre of each 'open' potato and pour any juice in as well. Sprinkle a little black pepper over each potato. Wrap *or* cover the potatoes and bake at 180°C/3550°F (Gas Mark 4) for 45 minutes. Serve immediately with other vegetables.

Carrot & Ginger Sauté

Serves 4

Value Per Portion:

Total Fat: .686 gm

Unsaturated Fat: .291 gm

Fibre: 2.278 gm

Calories: 87.93

Saturated Fat: .167 gm

Cholesterol: 0 mg

Sodium: 81.15 mg

3 cloves of Garlic
60ml (2 fl oz) apple juice
30g (1 oz) fresh ginger
450g (lb) carrots
1 bunch spring onions

Peel and chop the garlic and 'sauté' in the apple juice over a high heat. Thinly slice the ginger and carrots and add to the sauté, stirring frequently. Wash and trim the onions, slice them lengthwise and add to the sauté. However, do not stir them in yet – leave them on top of the carrots. Cover the pan and reduce the heat. Leave covered for 10 minutes then remove the cover, stir the vegetables well and serve with rice.

Spinach and Chickpea Mediterranean

Serves 4
Value Per Portion:
Total Fat: 7.372 gm
Unsaturated Fat: 5.324 gm
Fibre: 3.589 gm

Calories: 277.4
Saturated Fat: .889 gm
Cholesterol: 0 mg
Sodium: 104.5 mg

170g (6 oz) dry chickpeas
450g (1 lb) fresh spinach
15ml (1 tbsp) olive oil
3 cloves garlic
2 medium onions
5ml (1 tsp) caraway *or* cumin seeds
2.5ml (½ tsp) freshly ground black pepper

Wash, soak and cook the chickpeas. Wash, trim and drain the spinach. Heat the oil in a deep frying pan or saucepan and place over a medium flame. Finely chop the garlic and onion and sauté in the oil, stirring frequently. When the onion is tender, add the caraway and stir well. Add the cooked chickpeas and black pepper, cover the pan and cook for about 5 minutes. Roughly slice the spinach and place on top of the chickpeas. Cover the pan again and leave over a low flame for 10–15 minutes. Do not remove the cover. At the end of this time, stir the spinach into the chickpeas and serve immediately by itself, with rice or with steamed vegetables.

Tijuana Chili

Serves 4
Value Per Portion:
Total Fat: .845 gm
Unsaturated Fat: .408 gm
Fibre: 4.917 gm

Calories: 194.3
Saturated Fat: .099 gm
Cholesterol: 0 mg
Sodium: 699.3 mg

570ml (1 pint) water
1 medium onion
55g (2 oz) soya mince
140g (5 oz) tomato puree
1 × 400g (14 oz) tin chopped tomatoes
1.25–2.5ml (¼–½ tsp) chilli powder
1 × 450g (16 oz) tin kidney beans
30ml (2 tbsp) cider vinegar

Measure the water and tip a small amount into a deep saucepan. Place over a hugh flame and, when simmering, add the finely chopped onion. Sauté the onion for 3–5 minutes or until tender. Add the soya mince, tomato puree and the rest of the water and stir well. Reduce the heat and add the chilli powder and the beans, then cover the pan and leave to simmer for 25–30 minutes. 5 minutes before serving, add the vinegar and stir once again. Serve hot in bowls.

Shrimp-Stuffed Artichoke

Serves 1
Value Per Portion:
Total Fat: 1.381gm
Unsaturated Fat: .524gm
Fibre: 1.205gm

Calories: 94.63
Saturated Fat: .712gm
Cholesterol: 46.63mg
Sodium: 154.3mg

1 artichoke, cooked
6–8 shrimps, cooked and peeled
15ml (1 tbsp) finely chopped celery
15ml (1 tbsp) natural, low-fat yogurt
10ml (2 tsp) chopped mixed herbs

Carefully pull apart the artichoke leaves and scoop out the choke with a spoon. Mix the shrimps with the celery, yogurt and herbs, and fill the artichokes with the mixture.

Cauliflower Soufflés

Serves 4
Value Per Portion:
Total Fat: 4.564gm
Unsaturated Fat: 1.676gm
Fibre: .158gm

Calories: 152.1
Saturated Fat: 1.502gm
Cholesterol: 138.4mg
Sodium: 286.2mg

1 small cauliflower, trimmed of leaves and stalk
60ml (4 tbsp) whole wheat breadcrumbs
30ml (2 tbsp) plain, low-fat yogurt
15ml (1 tbsp) chopped fresh dill
2 eggs, separated
15ml (1 tbsp) grated Parmesan cheese
freshly ground black pepper

Preheat the oven to 375°F, 190°C, Gas 5. Cut the cauliflower into small florets, and cook in boiling water until just tender (keep the water for soup). Drain well and mash to a purée. Mix in the breadcrumbs, the yogurt, dill, egg yolks, and half the Parmesan cheese. Season to taste as well. Whisk the egg whites until stiff, then feld lightly into the cauliflower mixture. Spoon into four greased ramekin dishes, and sprinkle with the remaining cheese. Bake in the preheated oven for about 15–20 minutes until risen and golden. Serve immediately.

Poached Scallops with Yogurt Sauce

Serves 4
Value Per Portion:

Total Fat: 1.701gm	Calories: 100.5
Unsaturated Fat: .599gm	Saturated Fat: .777gm
Fibre: .94gm	Cholesterol: 14.38mg
	Sodium: 137.7mg

8 scallops, cleaned, but with their shells
1 crisp lettuce
Poaching stock
450ml (15 fl. oz) water
1 onion, peeled and roughly chopped
1 stalk celery, chopped
2 bay leaves
2–3 sprigs thyme or marjoram
6 black peppercorns
Sauce
5ml (1 tsp) Dijon mustard
285g (10 oz) natural, low-fat yogurt
15ml (1 tbsp) chopped fresh parsley
lemon juice
freshly ground black pepper

Wash the scallops in cold water, and clean four of the deep shells as well. Combine the poaching stock ingredients in a pan, bring to the boil slowly, then reduce to a simmer. Add the scallops and poach for about 8 minutes. Strain the scallops and leave to cool. Meanwhile, combine the sauce ingredients, adding lemon juice and seasoning to taste. Just before serving, shred the lettuce and use to make a nest on four plates. Pile the scallops in the middle of each nest, and spoon over the sauce.

Spicy Fish Kebabs

Serves 4
Value Per Portion:

Total Fat: 1.418gm	Calories: 150.2
Unsaturated Fat: .659gm	Saturated Fat: .393gm
Fibre: .013gm	Cholesterol: 96.62mg
	Sodium: 136.6mg

60ml (4 tbsp) plain, low-fat yoghurt
45ml (3 tbsp) lime juice
1 garlic clove, peeled and crushed
1 teaspoon ground coriander
1 thin slice fresh ginger, peeled and finely chopped
freshly ground black pepper
450g (1 lb) firm white fish, cut into 2.5cm (1 inch) cubes
12 large prawns, cooked and peeled
fresh coriander
lime wedges

Mix the yogurt with the lime juice, garlic, coriander, ginger and seasoning to taste. Stir the fish chunks and prawns into this and leave to chill for about 4 hours. Thread the drained pieces of fish and prawns evenly on to four skewers, and place on a baking sheet. Grill for about 5–6 minutes until the fish is cooked, brushing with leftover yogurt. Sprinkle with chopped fresh coriander and garnish with lime wedges.

Monkfish with Red Peppers

Serves 4
Value Per Portion:

Total Fat: 8.33gm	Calories: 172.8
Unsaturated Fat: 5.685gm	Saturated Fat: .945gm
Fibre: .96gm	Cholesterol: 28.35mg
	Sodium: 36.35mg

450g (1 lb) monkfish fillet, sliced
550ml (a scant pint) vegetable stock
4 garlic cloves, peeled and crushed
freshly ground black pepper
10ml (2 tsp) lemon juice
30ml (2 tbsp) olive oil
2 red peppers, cored, seeded and diced
1 crisp lettuce
15 ml (1 tbsp) chopped parsley

Steam the monkfish slices for about 3 minutes over the hot vegetable stock containing two of the crushed garlic cloves. Place the remaining garlic in a bowl, add a little seasoning to taste, the lemon juice and olive oil. Place the monkfish in this dressing, add the pepper dice, and leave at room temperature for a couple of hours. When cold, arrange in a bowl lined with lettuce leaves (or on nests of shredded lettuce leaves), and sprinkle with parsley.

Fish-Stuffed Spinach Leaves

Serves 4
Value Per Portion:

Total Fat: 4.363gm	Calories: 121.6
Unsaturated Fat: 3.216gm	Saturated Fat: .564gm
Fibre: .26gm	Cholesterol: 44.55mg
	Sodium: 534mg

115g (4 oz) fresh haddock, boned and skinned
170g (6 oz) crabmeat
1 egg white
lemon juice
freshly ground black pepper
5ml (1 tsp) olive oil
25g (1 oz) brown rice
60ml (2 fl. oz) vegetable stock
20 undamaged spinach or cabbage leaves, thick stalks removed

Place the haddock, crabmeat, egg white and 1 teaspoon lemon juice into the food processor, and blend until smooth. Add some seasoning to taste, then chill for about 30 minutes while you cook the rice. Heat the oil in a pan, stir in the rice, and then add the stock. Simmer, covered, until the stock has been absorbed (the rice will only be part cooked). Cool. Blanch the spinach leaves in boiling water, and drain and dry thoroughly. Mix the part-cooked rice into the fish mixture, and divide between the spinach leaves. Wrap up to form a parcel, and pack into a greased dish in one layer. Pour over a mixture of 15ml (1 tbsp) lemon juice and 15ml (1 tbsp) water, and place the dish in a roasting tin full of hot water. Bake, covered in an oven preheated to 350°F, 180°C, Gas 4 for about 1 hour. Serve hot or cold.

Lemon Chicken

Serves 4
Value Per Portion:
Total Fat: 5.18gm
Unsaturated Fat: 3.748gm
Fibre: .178gm

Calories: 129.1
Saturated Fat: .949gm
Cholesterol: 44mg
Sodium: 39.5mg

2 lemons, washed
1 small onion, thinly sliced
15ml (1 tbsp) olive oil
4 small chicken breasts, skinned and boned
30ml (2 tbsp) freshly chopped parsley
285ml (10 fl. oz) vegetable stock
freshly ground black pepper

Peel the rind thinly from one of the lemons and cut into tiny shreds. Halve both lemons and squeeze out the juice. Sauté the onion gently in the oil for a few minutes, then add the chicken breasts. Sauté until lightly browned on all sides. Add the parsley, stock and seasoning to the pan, along with the lemon juice, and cook gently covered, for about 20 minutes. Remove the chicken and keep warm while you reduce the sauce by boiling. Add the shred of lemon rind, warm through, then pour over the chicken.

Chicken En Papillote

Serves 4
Value Per Portion:
Total Fat: 1.4gm
Unsaturated Fat: .66gm
Fibre: .482gm

Calories: 133.9
Saturated Fat: .358gm
Cholesterol: 61.5mg
Sodium: 87.22mg

4 small chicken breasts, skinned and boned
50g (2 oz) carrots, scrubbed and cut into tiny strips
50g (2 oz) leeks, washed and cut into tiny strips
50g (2 oz) celery or celeriac, trimmed or peeled, then cut into tiny strips
100ml (4 fl. oz) vegetable stock
10ml (2 tsp) tarragon vinegar
freshly ground black pepper
15ml (1 tbsp) freshly chopped tarragon

Beat the chicken breasts to flatten them a little: Blanch the vegetable strips in boiling water for about a minute then drain well. Cut four pieces of good greaseproof paper large enough to completely enclose each chicken breast, and divide the vegetable strips between them. Place the chicken breasts on top, and sprinkle over the stock, vinegar and seasoning to taste. Close the packages well, then bake on a baking tray in an oven preheated to 400°F, 200°C, Gas 6 for about 20 minutes. When the packages are opened, sprinkle each with chopped tarragon.

Cooked Brown Rice

Serves 1
Value Per 340g (12oz) Cooked Portion:

Calories: 348

Total Fat: 1.8 gm
Unsaturated Fat: 0 gm
Fibre: 1–5 gm

Saturated Fat: 0 gm
Cholesterol: 0 mg
Sodium: 48 mg

Cooked Whole Wheat Pasta

Serves 1
Value Per 225g (8 oz) Serving:
Total Fat: 6.408 gm
Unsaturated Fat: 0 gm
Fibre: 10–20 gm

Calories: 206.5
Saturated Fat: 0 gm
Cholesterol: 0 mg
Sodium: no data

Whole Wheat Bread

Serves 1
Value Per 2 Slices:
Total Fat: 1.6 gm
Unsaturated Fat: 0 gm
Fibre: .4 gm

Calories: 122
Saturated Fat: .2 gm
Cholesterol: 0 mg
Sodium: 264 mg

SAUCES, DRESSINGS & SPREADS

Tangy Tomato Sauce

Serves 4
Value Per Portion:
Total Fat: .425 gm
Unsaturated Fat: .349 gm
Fibre: 1.582 gm

Calories: 152.2
Saturated Fat: .047 gm
Cholesterol: 0 mg
Sodium: 10.16 mg

140ml (5 fl oz) water
140ml (5 fl oz) cider vinegar
4 large prunes
1 lemon
140g (5 oz) tomato puree
2.5ml (½ tsp) ground coriander
5ml (1 tsp) paprika
5ml (1 tsp) freshly ground black pepper

Mix the water, vinegar and prunes together and leave to one side. Chop the lemon into small pieces and remove the pips. Empty the tomato puree into a small saucepan. Add the lemon pieces and the spices and stir well, then add the liquid with the softened prunes. Simmer the mixture over a low heat for 20 minutes, keeping it covered and stirring occasionally. Then remove from the heat, press the pips out of the prunes, remove the pips and leave the fruit in the sauce. You may leave the lemon pieces in if you like, as they are attractive. Serve this sauce hot over pasta, rice, vegetables or as the sauce for baked beans.

Poor Man's Guacamole

Serves 4
Value Per Portion:
Total Fat: 3.386 gm
Unsaturated Fat: .255 gm
Fibre: 2.984 gm

Calories: 161.8
Saturated Fat: .073 gm
Cholesterol: 0 mg
Sodium: 11.3 mg

455g (1 lb) cooked peas
285g (10 oz) soft tofu
1 small onion
2 cloves garlic
1 medium tomato
5ml (1 tsp) paprika

Mash the peas and tofu together in a bowl. Finely chop the onion, garlic and tomato and stir into the 'guacamole'. Add the paprika (or chilli powder if you prefer!), stir well, chill and serve with salad and toast.

Strong, Hot Dressing

Serves 4
Value Per Portion:
Total Fat: 7.1 gm
Unsaturated Fat: 5.523 gm
Fibre: .338 gm

Calories: 80.75
Saturated Fat: .904 gm
Cholesterol: 0 mg
Sodium: 17.3 mg

1 small fresh chilli
140ml (5 fl oz) cider vinegar
juice of 1 lemon
30ml (1 fl oz/2 tbsp) olive oil
5ml (1 tsp) dry mustard
30ml (1 fl oz/2 tbsp) soya milk

Chop the chilli, including its seeds, very finely and place in a jug or jam jar. Add the remaining ingredients to the jar and stir or shake very well. Serve immediately over salad, baked potato or pasta.

Easy Party Dip

Serves 4
Value Per Portion:
Total Fat: 3.425 gm
Unsaturated Fat: .161 gm
Fibre: .505 gm

Calories: 79.39
Saturated Fat: .028 gm
Cholesterol: 0 mg
Sodium: 39.77 mg

285g (10 oz) soft tofu
55g (2 oz) green olives
2 spring onions
1 eating apple
10ml (2 tsp) dill or caraway seeds

Mash the tofu in a serving bowl. Finely chop the olives and onions and stir into the tofu. Peel and grate the apple into the mixture. Add the dill seed and and stir the mixture very well. Chill for 30 minutes before serving.

All Salad Dresing

Serves 4
Value Per Portion:
Total Fat: 7.194 gm
Unsaturated Fat: 5.772 gm
Fibre: .041 gm

Calories: 67.67
Saturated Fat: .946 gm
Cholesterol: 0 mg
Sodium: 32.38 mg

3 cloves of garlic
30ml (1 fl oz) oil
90ml (3 fl oz) cider vinegar
10ml (2 tsp) wet mustard
2.5ml (½ tsp) dried parsley *or* mixed sweet herbs

Chop or crush the garlic into a jug or jar. Add the other ingredients and shake or stir the mixture very well. Serve over any salad.

Silky Peanut Sauce

Serves 4
Value Per Portion:
Total Fat: 2.055 gm
Unsaturated Fat: 1.605 gm
Fibre: .158 gm

Calories: 29.75
Saturated Fat: .343 gm
Cholesterol: 0 mg
Sodium: 1.25 mg

15ml (1 tbsp) unsalted crunchy peanut butter
2 cloves garlic
juice of 1 lemon
285ml (10 fl oz) water

Measure the peanut butter into a small saucepan and place over a medium heat. Finely chop the garlic and add to the peanut butter. Stir often. When the peanut butter is melted, add the lemon juice. Stir well and gradually add the water, stirring after each addition. Reduce the heat and keep covered for 5–10 minutes. Serve hot with rice or vegetables.

Versatile Fennel Sauce

Serves 4
Value Per Portion:
Total Fat: .223 gm
Unsaturated Fat: .129 gm
Fibre: .548 gm

Calories: 28.75
Saturated Fat: .032 gm
Cholesterol: 0 mg
Sodium: 24.5 mg

1 large sweet fennel
1 green eating apple
juice of 1 lemon
2.5ml (½ tsp) ground coriander

Wash and trim the fennel and apple and cut into small chunks. Place in a food processor. Add the lemon juice and the coriander to the processor and puree all the ingredients together to a fine consistency. Serve chilled as a dip for raw vegetables, a garnish in soups or as salad dressing.

Coriander & Lentil Pâté

Serves 4
Value Per Portion:
Total Fat: .733 gm
Unsaturated Fat: .204 gm
Fibre: 1.827 gm

Calories: 95.54
Saturated Fat: .125 gm
Cholesterol: 0 mg
Sodium: 54.65 mg

225g (8 oz) dried red lentils
550–710ml (1–1¼ pint) water
50g (2 oz) porridge oats
50g (2 oz) rice flakes
5ml (1 tsp) ground black pepper *or* paprika
2.5ml (½ tsp) ground ginger
30g (1 oz) fresh coriander leaves

Wash and drain the lentils, add the clean water and bring to a soft boil over a medium heat. Reduce the heat, cover and simmer for 30 minutes, stirring often. Add oats, rice flakes, pepper and ginger and cook for another 5–10 minutes. Wash and chop the coriander. Remove the pâté from the heat, stir in the coriander and spoon into a serving dish. Allow the pâté to cool, then chill or serve immediately.

BREAKFASTS & BEVERAGES

Easy Fruit Muesli

Serves 4
Value Per Portion:
Total Fat: 9.036 gm
Unsaturated Fat: 6.931 gm
Fibre: 6.444 gm

Calories: 507.7
Saturated Fat: 1.156 gm
Cholesterol: 0 mg
Sodium: 15.97 mg

50g (2 oz) dried dates
50g (2 oz) dried figs
1 eating apple
1 banana
50g (2 oz) raisins

50g (2 oz) sunflower seeds
300ml (10 fl oz) apple juice
50g (2 oz) rolled oats
2.5ml (½ tsp) cinnamon

Wash and chop the dates, figs and apple. Peel and slice the banana; mix all the fruit with the raisins, seeds and applie juice ina large bowl. Add the oats and cinnamon and stir well. Allow to sit for 10 minutes then serve in small bowls.

Breakfast Melon

Serves 4
Value Per Portion:
Total Fat: 7.967 gm
Unsaturated Fat: 6.458 gm
Fibre: 2.582 gm

Calories: 265.4
Saturated Fat: .793 gm
Cholesterol: 0 mg
Sodium: 35.69 mg

2 satsumas *or* mandarins
55g (2 oz) raisins *or* sultanas
55g (2 oz) hazelnuts *or* slivered almonds
140ml (5 fl oz) orange juice
1 whole honeydew melon

Divide the satsumas into segments and place them in a bowl with the raisins, hazelnuts and orange juice. Stir well and leave to soak for 5–10 minutes. Cut the melon into four and scoop out the seeds. Spoon the fruit mixture onto the melon quarters. Serve immediately.

Quick Sweet Porridge

Serves 4
Value Per Portion:
Total Fat: 24.89 gm
Unsaturated Fat: 3.807 gm
Fibre: 4.226 gm

Calories: 582.8
Saturated Fat: .891 gm
Cholesterol: 0 mg
Sodium: 44.05 mg

55g (2 oz) porridge oats (per person)
30g (1 oz) raisins or sultanas (p.p.)
285ml (½ pint) soya milk

Measure all the ingredients into a small saucepan and place over a low heat. Stir frequently as the mixture thickens and leave to cook for 7–10 minutes. Serve hot with a sprinkling of ground cinnamon.

Superior Muesli

Serves 4
Value Per Portion:
Total Fat: 20.775 gm
Unsaturated Fat: 13.57 gm
Fibre: 1.698 gm

Calories: 383.2
Saturated Fat: 1.70 gm
Cholesterol: 0 mg
Sodium: 8.755 mg

55g (2 oz) rolled oats (p.p. or for 2 p.)
30g (1 oz) barley flakes
30g (1 oz) raisins or sultanas
30g (1 oz) chopped dried date
30g (1 oz) sunflower seeds
30g (1 oz) walnut pieces
285ml (½ pint) soya milk *or* fruit juice

Mix all the dry ingredients together in a large breakfast bowl and pour the milk or juice over them. Leave to sit five minutes before eating.

Traditional Mixed Grill

Serves 4
Value Per Portion:
Total Fat: 12.64 gm
Unsaturated Fat: .561 gm
Fibre: 9.872 gm

Calories: 445.1
Saturated Fat: .351 gm
Cholesterol: 0 mg
Sodium: 868 mg

1 vegetarian burger (p.p.)
2 medium tomatoes, halved
55g (2 oz) mushrooms
2 slices whole wheat bread
85g (3 oz) sugarless baked beans
30ml (2 tbsp) tomato ketchp *or* brown sauce

Place the burger under a hot grill with the tomatoes and mush-rooms. Toast the breat and heat the baked beans. Pour the beans over one piece of toast if you like, add the sauce and serve.

Thick Banana Milkshake

Serves 4
Value Per Portion:
Total Fat: 8.68 gm
Unsaturated Fat: .197 gm
Fibre: .815 gm

Calories: 250.2
Saturated Fat: .276 gm
Cholesterol: 0 mg
Sodium: 10.7 mg

2–3 ripe bananas
570ml (1 pint) soya milk
2.5ml (½ tsp) ground allspice

Peel the bananas and break them into a large blender. Add the milk and allspice and whisk to a thick, even consistency. Serve immediately or chill for 10 minutes. Garnish with a sprig of rosemary or cinnamon stick

Sharp Citrus Drink

Serves 4
Value Per Portion:
Total Fat: .282 gm
Unsaturated Fat: .105 gm
Fibre: .083 gm

Calories: 109.9
Saturated Fat: .936 gm
Cholesterol: 0 mg
Sodium: 3 mg

2 grapefruits
2 large oranges
2 lemons
1 lime
1 sprig of fresh mint
570ml (1 pint) sparkling mineral water

Squeeze the fruits and pour their juices together into a large serving jug. Coarsely chop the mint and add to the juice, then pour the mineral water slowly over the juice. Stir gently, chill and serve.

Pure Almond Milk

Serves 4
Value Per Portion:
Total Fat: 29.84 gm
Unsaturated Fat: 25.632 gm
Fibre: 1.3 gm

Calories: 332
Saturated Fat: 2.828 gm
Cholesterol: 0 mg
Sodium: 6 mg

115 (4 oz) whole shelled almonds
850 (1.5 pints) very cold water

Measure the almonds into a mixing bowl and cover them with
tepid water. Leave them to soak overnight, or for 8–12 hours.
Drain and rinse the soaked almonds and remove their skins.
This is made easier if you pour a little boiling water over the
soaked almonds. Put the peeled almonds in a food processor
with the cold water. Puree to a very fine, very smooth consistency. Strain the milk through cheesecloth or a paper coffee filter
into a jug. Allow 10–15 minutes for the milk to finish filtering.
Serve this pure white milk immediately. use the almond pulp in
baking if you wish.

Hot Carob Comforter

Serves 4
Value Per Portion: Calories: 160.6
Total Fat: 9.938 gm   Saturated Fat: .001 gm
Unsaturated Fat: .004 gm   Cholesterol: 0 mg
Fibre: .06 gm   Sodium: 15.1 mg

200ml (7 fl oz) soya milk (pp)
15ml (1 tbsp) powdered carob

Make as you would hot chocolate. Pour most of the milk into
a small saucepan and place over a low heat. Stir the carob into
the remaining milk until smooth. Pour the carob mixture into
the warm milk and, using a wire whisk, stir to a froth until the
milk is hot. Pour immediately into a mug and serve.

Fruit Juices

Apple

Serves 1
Value Per ½ pint (10 fl. oz)   Calories: 145
Portion:
Total Fat: .35 gm   Saturated Fat: .059 gm
Unsaturated Fat: .118 gm   Cholesterol: 0 mg
Fibre: .65 gm   Sodium: 8.75 mg

Orange

Serves 1
Value Per ½ pint (10 fl oz) Portion:

Calories: 138.8

Total Fat: .635 gm
Unsaturated Fat: .235 gm
Fibre: .313 gm

Saturated Fat: .075 gm
Cholesterol: 0 mg
Sodium: 2.5 mg

Grapefruit

Serves 1
Value Per ½ pint (10 fl oz) Portion:

Calories: 120

Total Fat: .313 gm
Unsaturated Fat: .114 gm
Fibre: .313 gm

Saturated Fat: .044 gm
Cholesterol: 0 mg
Sodium: 2.5 mg

Pineapple

Serves 1
Value Per ½ pint (10 fl oz) Portion:

Calories: 173.8

Total Fat: .25 gm
Unsaturated Fat: .117 gm
Fibre: .313 gm

Saturated Fat: .016 gm
Cholesterol: 0 mg
Sodium: 2.5 mg

Grape

Serves 1
Value Per ½ pint. (10 fl oz) Portion:

Calories: 193.8

Total Fat: .238 gm
Unsaturated Fat: .08 gm
Fibre: .313 gm

Saturated Fat: .079 gm
Cholesterol: 0 mg
Sodium: 8.75 mg

Herbal Teas

Serves 1
Value Per ½ pint (10 fl oz) Portion:

Calories: 1.59

Total Fat: .023 gm
Unsaturated Fat: .017 gm
Fibre: 0 gm

Saturated Fat: .006 gm
Cholesterol: 0 mg
Sodium: 3.18 mg

DESSERTS & SNACKS

Hot Fruit Compote

Serves 4
Value Per Portion:
Total Fat: .481 gm
Unsaturated Fat: .165 gm
Fibre: .954 gm

Calories: 152.7
Saturated Fat: .078 gm
Cholesterol: 0 mg
Sodium: 4.813 mg

2 grapefruit
2 oranges
1 lemon
1 tart apple
50g (2 oz) raisins

For the Sauce
140ml (5 fl oz) red wine
1.25l (¼ tsp) ground cloves
1.25ml (¼ tsp) ground cinnamon

Carefully peel and section the citrus fruits and place in a shallow casserole dish. Chop the apple, add the apple and raisins to the citrus fruits and stir well. Prepare the sauce by mixing the wine and spices together in a jug. Pour this over the fruit and allow it to soak for 10 minutes. Stir again. Warm the oven to 170°C/ 325°F (Gas Mark 3). Cover the compote and bake for 20 minutes. Serve immediately, pouring a little of the hot sauce over each serving.

Spicy Oat Cake

Serves 4
Value Per Portion:
Total Fat: 6.292 gm
Unsaturated Fat: 4.873 gm
Fibre: 2.584 gm

Calories: 210.8
Saturated Fat: .827 gm
Cholesterol: 0 mg
Sodium: 68.3 mg

2 tart apples
55g (2 oz) whole wheat flour
115g (4 oz) rolled oats
2.5ml (½ tsp) ground cinnamon
1.25ml (¼ tsp) ground cloves
5ml (1 tsp) baking powder
285 ml (10 fl oz) water
15ml (1 tbsp) oil

Warm the oven to 160°C/300°F (Gas Mark 3) and lightly oil a 20cm (8 inch) cake tin. Peel and finely chop the apples and mix them with the dry ingredients in a mixing bowl. Stir the water and oil together and pour this liquid into the dry mix. Stir well, adding a little more water if necessary to give a smooth, moist batter. Spoon the batter into the cake tin, spread evenly to the corners and bake for 25–30 minutes. Cool for 15 minutes, then remove from the tin and cool on a rack.

Slice & Serve Bars

Serves 4
Value Per Portion: Calories: 876
Total Fat: 21.15 gm   Saturated Fat: 2.927 gm
Unsaturated Fat: 14.948 gm   Cholesterol: 0 mg
Fibre: 4.77 gm   Sodium: 259 mg

225g (8 oz) whole wheat flour
55g (2 oz) rolled oats
55g (2 oz) raisins *or* sultanas
5ml (1 tsp) baking powder
2.5ml (½ tsp) ground cinnamon *or* allspice
15ml (1 tbsp) oil
5ml (1 tsp) natural vanilla essence
140ml (5 fl oz) water

Warm the oven to 160°C/300°F (Gas Mark 3) and lightly oil a 20cm (8 inch) cake tin. Mix the first five ingredients together in a mixing bowl. Mix the oil, essence and water, add to the dry mix and stir well. Spoon the batter evenly into the cake tin and bake for 25 minutes. Allow to cool, then slice and serve.

Heavenly Cake

Serves 4
Value Per Portion: Calories: 1626
Total Fat: 70.93 gm   Saturated Fat: 9.195 gm
Unsaturated Fat: 52.01 gm   Cholesterol: 0 mg
Fibre: 19.53 gm   Sodium: 288 mg

115g (4 oz) whole-wheat flour
115g (4 oz) rolled oats
55g (2 oz) oat bran
115g (4 oz) raisins or sultanas

2.5ml (½ tsp) ground cinnamon
2.5ml (½ tsp) ground cloves
5ml (1 tsp) baking powder
285ml (10 fl oz) water OR fruit juice
30ml (1 fl oz/2 tbsp) oil

Pre-heat the oven to 180°C/350°F (Gas Mark 4) and lightly oil a 20cm (8 inch) baking tin. Mix the dry ingredients together in a large mixing bowl. Measure the fruit juice and oil together into a jug and pour gradually into the dry mix, stirring well after each addition. Spread the better evenly into the cake tin and bake for 30 minutes. Cool slightly before removing it from the tin. Cool on a wire rack.

Superlative Cake

Serves 4
Value Per Portion:
Total Fat: 73.73 gm
Unsaturated Fat: 56.74gm
Fibre: 11.63 gm

Calories: 2544
Saturated Fat: 8.659 gm
Cholesterol: 0 mg
Sodium: 316.6 mg

455g (1 lb) whole-wheat flour
115g (4 oz) rolled oats
5ml (1 tsp) baking powder
2.5ml (½ tsp) ground ginger
55g (2 oz) almond flakes
225g (8 oz) dried currants
55g (2 oz) citrus peel
30ml (1 fl oz/2 tbsp) oil
570ml (1 pint) fruit juice

Mix the first five ingredients together in a large mixing bowl. Mix the remaining ingredients together in a jug and leave to one side for 10 minutes. Pre-heat the oven to 180°C/350°F (Gas Mark 4) and lightly oil a 23cm × 33cm (9 inch × 134 inch) cake tin. Stir the moist ingredidents into the dry ingredients. Spoon the batter into the cake tin and bake for 30 minutes. Cool on a wire rack before slicing.

Delicious Stuffed Dates

Serves 4
Value Per Portion:
Total Fat: 84.42 gm
Unsaturated Fat: 60.81 gm
Fibre: 15.75 gm

Calories: 2180
Saturated Fat: 6.364 gm
Cholesterol: 0 mg
Sodium: 42.8mg

455g (1 lb) fresh dates
285g (10 oz) soft tofu
5ml (1 tsp) freshly ground coriander
115g (4 oz) walnut halves

Wash the dates, then slice each one in half lengthwise and remove the stone. Do not cut all the way through the dates. Blend the tofu and coriander into a smooth paste and spoon a little into each open date. Press a walnut half onto the filling and place the date on a serving plate. Continue in this way until all the dates are filled. Chill before serving.

Tofu Cheese and Biscuits

Serves 4
Value Per Portion:
Total Fat: 23.12 gm
Unsaturated Fat: .037 gm
Fibre: .442 gm *

Calories: 449.5
Saturated Fat: 2.412 gm
Cholesterol: 0 mg
Sodium: 561. mg

285g (10 oz) firm tofu
15ml (1 tbsp) mild mustard
15ml (1 tbsp) soya milk
2 spring onions *or* 15ml (1 tbsp) chives
16 matzos

Break the tofu into a blender, add the mustard and the milk and puree to a smooth consistency. Add a little more milk for a softer cheese. Spoon the mixture into the serving bowl and add the finely chopped onion or chives. Stir well and serve immediately or chill for 30 minutes. Spread a little on each of the matzos. NOTE: A single cracker has only 17 calories and .05 grams of fat. Matzos are made without added salt or fat.

Additional Suggestions for snacks and desserts:

- A plate of raw vegetables (crudites) served with a selection of dips, sauces and pâté from the previous section is a healthy snack or late dessert.
- A bowl of raw fruit or a salad made from a mixture of fresh fruit. Serve with a little chilled fruit juice that has been flavoured with ground cinnamon or allspice.
- A selection of whole nuts, still in their shells, is a nutritiucutritious snack or dessert that is impossible to rush through — the shelling process is usually so slow that most people only eat twelve to fifteen nuts.

APPENDIX

Anemia – a shortage of red blood cells, and therefore haemoglobin, in your blood.

Aneurysm – a weak point in the wall of an artery which bulges and may burst, or rupture

Angina (pectoris) – a distinct, gripping pain in the chest indicating that the muscle of your heart is not receiving enough oxygen

Artery – the channel, or vessel, which carries blood away from your heart

Atheroma – from the Greek meaing 'porridge'. Atheroma is the mixture of fat, blood and calcium which builds up in deposits along the artery walls

Atherosclerosis – a hardening and narrowing of the artieres due to build up of atheroma

Atrium (plura = atria) – the 'waiting rooms' of your heart. The two upper chambers of your heart which collect blood prior to it being pumped out of the heart again

Calcification – a feature of advanced atherosclerosis, the addition of calcium to the deposits (atheroma) causing them to harden

Calorie – a measure of a unit of heart or energy. Food converts into energy and the amount of energy each food gives is measured in calories

Carbon Monoxide – a very poisonous gas present in car exhaust and cigarette smoke

Carboxy-haemoglobin – the substance which takes the place of oxygen in the red blood cell in those who smoke. Carbon monoxide combines with haemoglobin to create carboxy-haemoglobin

Cardiac – having to do with the heart

Cardiovascular – having to do with the heart and the blood vessels

Cerebrovascular – having to do with the brain and the blood vessels. In particular with the supply of blood to the brain.

Cholesterol – a fatty substance found in all animal fats.

Coronary – relating to the heart. Some people say 'he's had a coronary' when referring to someone who has had a heart attack.

Coronary Heart Disease – a term used to describe the group of symptoms which result from diseased coronary arteries. These include angina, heart attack and sudden death.

Coronary Thrombosis – a coronary artery blocked by a blood clot

Diastole – the lowest blood pressure reading. From the point in your heart beat when the heart muscle is relaxed

Embolism – blockage of an artery (usually quite sudden) by a break-away atheroma deposit, blood clot or foreign body

Erythrocytes – red blood cells

Fatty Acid – the substances in fat that give it its unique flavour, texture and melting point

Glucose – also called blood sugar, this is the final product from your body's breakdown of carbohydrate food

Haemoglobin – the pigment of your red blood cells, containing iron, which carries oxygen and carbon dioxide

Hardening of the arteries – the process of atherosclerosis with calcification

Heart Attack – see myocardial infarction

Hemorrhage – an abnormal discharge of blood, internally or externally

Hormone – a chemical secreted by your glands which travels through your tissue fluid to an organ where it triggers a specific effect on your metabolism

Hypertension – abnormally high blood pressure

Infarct – an area of dead tissue, or scar tissue. An infarction is the death of tissue due to loss of oxygen supply.

Ischaemic (heart disease) – having to do with lack of blood supply, therefore causing lack of oxygen supply

Leucocytes – white blood cells

Lipid – a fat substance

Metabolism – the chemical process of assimilating food by turning it into energy and substances which will repair and replace body tissues. Your metabolism includes all of the stages and features of this process

Myocardial infarction – also known as heart attack. The death of heart muscle after its supply of blood, and therefore oxygen, has been interrupted

Myocardium – the heart muscle itself. The muscle wall of the heart

Obesity – the state of being excessively overweight

Serum – as in serum cholesterol, that measured in the blood

Stroke – a cerebrovascular accident. Damage in an area of brain due to the blockage of rupture of a blood vessel in the brain

Systole – the highest blood pressure reading. From the point in your heart beat when your heart muscle is contracting, or pumping

Thrombus (thrombosis) – a blood clot. Thrombosis is the formation of a blood clot

Tissue – cells of a particular kind which group together for a specific function, i.e. muscle tissue, skin tissue, bone tissue.

Toxic – having the effect of a poison. The amount of a substance which may be toxic will vary depending on individual tolerances for it

Vascular – having to do with blood vessels blood supply

Veins – blood vessels or channels that return blood to the heart

Ventricle (plural = ventricles) – the two lower chambers of the heart which pump blood out of the heart into the arteries.

FURTHER READING

Exercise for the Over-50s, Dr. Russell Gibbs, Jill Norman Ltd., 1981

Losing Weight Naturally, Caroline LaPorte, Century Hutchinson Ltd., London 1989

Relaxation East and West: A Manual of Poised Living, James Hewitt, Rider, London 1982

Tempeh Cookery, Colleen Pride.

Tofu Cookery, Louise Hagler

Vegan Nutrition, Dr. Michael A. Klaper, Vegan Society Publications, Oxford 1988

Vegan Nutrition, Gill Langley, Vegan Society Publications, Oxford 1988

Why You Don't Need Meat, Peter Cox, Thorsons Publishers Ltd, Wellingborough 1986

USEFUL ADDRESSES

Action on Smoking and Health (ASH), 5–11 Mortimer Street, London W1N 7RJ, tel: 01–637–9643

British Cardiac Society, 7 St Andrew's Place, London NW1: 01–486–6430

British Heart Foundation, 102 Gloucester Place, London W1H 4DH, tel: 01–953–0185 NOTE: there are eleven regional offices for the BHF. Please look in your phone directory for that nearest to you.

British Holistic Medical Association, 179 Gloucester Place, London NW1 6DX tel: 01–262–5299

British Wheel of Yoga, 80 Leckhampton Road, Cheltenham, Gloucestershire GL53 0BN

The Coronary Artery Disease Research Association (COROA), Tavistock House North, Tavistock Square, London WC1H 9TH, tel: 01–387–9779

Coronary Prevention Group, 60 Great Ormond Street, London WC1N 3HR, tel: 01–833–3687

Coronary Prevention in Children Project, Exeter Health Authority, Exeter

Greater London Alcohol Advisory Service (GLASS), 146 Queen Victoria Street, London EC4V 4BX, tel: 01–248 8406

The Health Education Authority, 78 New Oxford Street, London WC1A 1AH, tel: 01–631–0930

The Keep Fit Association, National Secretary, 16 Upper Woburn Place, London WC1H 0QG, tel: 01–387–4349

Northern Ireland ASH, c/o The Ulster Cancer Foundation, 40 Eglantine Avenue, Belfast BT9 6DX

Northern Ireland Coronary Prevention Group, Bryson House, 28 Bedford Street, Belfast BT2 7FJ

Scottish ASH, Royal College of Physicians, 9 Queen's Street, Edinburgh EH2 1JQ

Scottish Health Eduction Group, health Education Centre, Woodburn House, Canaan Lane, Edinburgh EH10 4SG

The Vegan Society, 33–35 George Street, Oxford OX1 2AX, tel: 0865–722166

The Women's League of Health and Beauty, 18 Charing Cross Road, London WC2 0HR, tel: 01–240–8456

NOTE: The following organizations each have regional offices, please look in your phone book for that nearest to you. Ring or write for advice on first aid courses that may help you save the life of someone having a heart attack.

Ambu International, Head Office, Charlton Road, Midsomer Norton, Bath BA3 4DR

The British Red Cross Society, Head Office, 9 Grosvenor Crescent, London SW1X 7EJ

The Royal Life-saving Society, Head Office, Mountbatten House, Studley, Warwickshire

St. Andrew's Ambulance Association, Head Office, Milton Street, Glasgow G4 0HR

St. John's Ambulance, Head Office, 1 Grosvenor Crescent, London SW1X 7EF, tel: 01–235–5231

Index